THE
EVERYTHING
GUIDE TO
THE ACID REFLUX DIET

Dear Reader,

I'm glad you've decided to read *The Everything® Guide to the Acid Reflux Diet*. As with anything I write, I've put forth my best effort in giving you a book that is easy to read, chock-full of useful nuggets of knowledge, and most importantly, contains information that can help you not only treat your acid reflux, but prevent it. That's because I'm not like your regular run-of-the-mill family doc, even though I'm currently the Chairman and Medical Director of the Michigan State University College of Osteopathic Medicine Family & Community Medicine Department. I'm residency trained and board certified in preventive medicine, public health, and integrative medicine, so to me, helping my patients—and you, my readers—prevent an illness or disease is just as important to me—if not more so—than treating the disease itself. Yes, I know that's pretty radical thinking in this day and age of insurance-driven healthcare that is government mandated and regulated, but that's okay; I'm very comfortable working outside the mainstream if that's what it takes to give the best care and information to both my patients and you!

Edward Rosick, DO, MPH, DABIHM

Welcome to the EVERYTHING® Series!

These handy, accessible books give you all you need to tackle a difficult project, gain a new hobby, comprehend a fascinating topic, prepare for an exam, or even brush up on something you learned back in school but have since forgotten.

You can choose to read an Everything® book from cover to cover or just pick out the information you want from our four useful boxes: e-questions, e-facts, e-alerts, and e-ssentials.

We give you everything you need to know on the subject, but throw in a lot of fun stuff along the way, too.

We now have more than 400 Everything® books in print, spanning such wide-ranging categories as weddings, pregnancy, cooking, music instruction, foreign language, crafts, pets, New Age, and so much more. When you're done reading them all, you can finally say you know Everything®!

QUESTION

Answers to common questions

FACT

Important snippets of information

ALERT

Urgent warnings

ESSENTIAL

Quick handy tips

PUBLISHER Karen Cooper

MANAGING EDITOR, EVERYTHING® SERIES Lisa Laing

COPY CHIEF Casey Ebert

ASSISTANT PRODUCTION EDITOR Alex Guarco

ACQUISITIONS EDITOR Hillary Thompson

SENIOR DEVELOPMENT EDITOR Brett Palana-Shanahan

EVERYTHING® SERIES COVER DESIGNER Erin Alexander

Visit the entire Everything® series at *www.everything.com*

THE EVERYTHING® GUIDE TO THE ACID REFLUX DIET

Manage your symptoms, relieve pain,
and heal your acid reflux naturally

Edward R. Rosick, DO, MPH, DABIHM

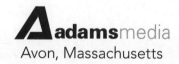

Adams media
Avon, Massachusetts

An Everything® Series Book.
Everything® and everything.com® are registered trademarks of F+W Media, Inc.

Published by
Adams Media, a division of F+W Media, Inc.
57 Littlefield Street, Avon, MA 02322. U.S.A.
www.adamsmedia.com

Contains material adapted and abridged from *The Everything® Vegetarian Cookbook* by Jay Weinstein, copyright © 2002 by F+W Media, Inc., ISBN 10: 1-58062-640-8, ISBN 13: 978-1-58062-640-8; *The Everything® Gluten-Free Cookbook* by Rick Marx and Nancy T. Maar, copyright © 2006 by F+W Media, Inc., ISBN 10: 1-59337-394-5, ISBN 13: 978-1-59337-394-8; *The Everything® Food Allergy Cookbook* by Linda Larsen, copyright © 2008 by F+W Media, Inc., ISBN 10: 1-59869-560-6, ISBN 13: 978-1-59869-560-1; *The Everything® Slow Cooker Cookbook, 2nd Edition* by Pamela Rice Hahn, copyright © 2009, 2002 by F+W Media, Inc., ISBN 10: 1-59869-977-6, ISBN 13: 978-1-59869-977-7; *The Everything® Glycemic Index Cookbook, 2nd Edition* by LeeAnn Smith Weintraub, copyright © 2010, 2006 by F+W Media, Inc., ISBN 10: 1-4405-0584-5, ISBN 13: 978-1-4405-0584-3; *The Everything® Juicing Book* by Carole Jacobs and Patrice Johnson with Nicole Cormier, copyright © 2010 by F+W Media, Inc., ISBN 10: 1-4405-0326-5, ISBN 13: 978-1-4405-0326-9; *The Everything® Green Smoothies Book* by Britt Brandon, copyright © 2011 by F+W Media, Inc., ISBN 10: 1-4405-2564-1, ISBN 13: 978-1-4405-2564-3; *The Everything® Gluten-Free Slow Cooker* by Carrie S. Forbes, copyright © 2012 by F+W Media, Inc., ISBN 10: 1-4405-3366-0, ISBN 13: 978-1-4405-3366-2; *The Everything® Vegetarian Slow Cooker Cookbook* by Amy Snyder and Justin Snyder, copyright © 2012 by F+W Media, Inc., ISBN 10: 1-4405-2858-6, ISBN 13: 978-1-4405-2858-3; *The Everything® Eating Clean Cookbook* by Britt Brandon, copyright © 2012 by F+W Media, Inc., ISBN 10: 1-4405-2999-X, ISBN 13: 978-1-4405-2999-3; and *The Everything® Gluten-Free Baking Cookbook* by Carrie S. Forbes, copyright © 2013 by F+W Media, Inc., ISBN 10: 1-4405-6486-8, ISBN 13: 978-1-4405-6486-4.

ISBN 10: 1-4405-8626-8
ISBN 13: 978-1-4405-8626-2
eISBN 10: 1-4405-8627-6
eISBN 13: 978-1-4405-8627-9

Printed in the United States of America.

10   9   8   7   6   5   4   3   2   1

Library of Congress Cataloging-in-Publication Data

Rosick, Edward R.
  Everything guide to the acid reflux diet / Edward R. Rosick, DO, MPH, DABIHM.
      pages cm
  Includes bibliographical references and index.
  ISBN 978-1-4405-8626-2 (pb) – ISBN 1-4405-8626-8 (pb) – ISBN 978-1-4405-8627-9 (ebook) – ISBN 1-4405-8627-6 (ebook)
  1. Gastroesophageal reflux–Popular works. 2. Gastroesophageal reflux–Diet therapy. 3. Gastroesophageal reflux–Diet therapy–Recipes. I. Title.
  RC815.7.R598 2015
  641.5'63–dc23

                               2014046373

Contents

Introduction

ACID REFLUX. GASTROESOPHAGEAL REFLUX disease. These and other terms describe a condition in which acid from the stomach—where it's supposed to be—goes into the esophagus—where it's *not* supposed to be—and from there the story goes rapidly downhill. Because of that acid in the esophagus, people who suffer from acid reflux can have a number of symptoms including heartburn, nausea, coughing, and chest pain. And while those symptoms can range from being an occasional annoyance to a debilitating chronic condition, there are more deadly consequences of untreated acid reflux, such as esophageal cancer. That last fact alone makes a book on acid reflux well worth writing and reading.

Acid reflux isn't just something that strikes a person here or there; the fact of the matter is that 60 percent of the U.S. adult population will suffer from acid reflux within a yearly timeframe, while 20–30 percent of the adult population will suffer weekly. In a population of over 300 million people, those facts make acid reflux one of the most common diagnoses seen in doctors' offices every day. But acid reflux is not just seen and treated in physicians' offices; studies have shown that hospitalizations due to acid reflux rose over 100 percent in just an 8-year period between 1996 and 2004. Some of those hospitalizations were due to esophageal cancer—a cancer linked to untreated or undertreated acid reflux—which has been increasing in incidence in the United States despite the hundreds of billions of dollars spent on the war on cancer.

This book, *The Everything® Guide to the Acid Reflux Diet*, will give you the tools you need in order to talk to your physician about acid reflux. This book will help you understand and prevent acid reflux, and gain knowledge about how acid reflux is treated. While some books on medical and health subjects are dry and boring, *The Everything® Guide to the Acid Reflux Diet* will present you with up-to-date information backed up by the latest studies in an easy-to-read voice.

In Chapter 1, you'll learn how the digestive system works, not in the dry, scholarly tone of a medical school textbook, but rather in an interesting and engaging manner; then, you'll be able to use that information to understand the basic facts about acid reflux that follow. In Chapter 2, you will learn how foods and beverages can make acid reflux worse (as well as what ones can make it better); in addition, you'll learn new information on how acid reflux may very well be related to gluten sensitivity, all backed up by recent scientific studies.

Chapter 3 delves into areas that many physicians don't cover with their patients, with one of those being stress and how it can negatively impact health, including causing acid reflux, and how you can manage that stress. Chapter 3 also examines the ways in which obesity has fueled the rise in acid reflux and provides common-sense tips you can use to curb unhealthy eating patterns both at home and out on the town.

In Chapter 4, you'll learn about the medications that are commonly, as well as not-so-commonly, used to treat acid reflux, and gain the knowledge to help you decide what pharmaceutical drugs you might wish to discuss with your doctor in regard to treatment. Chapter 5 focuses on integrative and alternative therapies for acid reflux, looking at some nonconventional treatments in a fun but informative matter, all the while keeping things grounded with the latest studies. Chapter 6 presents the final option—surgery—for those people for whom lifestyle changes, medications, and alternative therapies have failed to adequately treat their acid reflux. Finally, this book ends with a number of delicious, nutritious, and easy to make recipes that are not only healthy but have been especially chosen for people with acid reflux.

In conclusion, *The Everything® Guide to the Acid Reflux Diet* is a book that will inform, entertain, and give practical, useful, and understandable knowledge to anyone who suffers from acid reflux—or lives with someone who has acid reflux—so that this common disease can not just be treated, but prevented.

The ABCs of Acid Reflux

Welcome to Chapter 1. Here you'll learn about the digestive system—that part of your body that turns food into energy. During this process there are times when things sometimes go wrong, with one of the most common things being acid reflux. Acid reflux is a devious foe because it can masquerade as a variety of other problems, leading many people to delay getting treatment. This delay can cause a multitude of problems some of which can be life threatening. This chapter will explain all the parts of the digestive system so you can see what is going on in your body when acid reflux strikes.

Anatomy of the Digestive Tract

The human body is an amazing thing. It is incredible to think about how two single cells can come together and combine to make organisms that can think, sing, dance, and send rockets to the edge of our solar system. Yet for all the accomplishments of the human race throughout the ages, we are still captive to some basic physiological facts, and one of those is how to produce energy to power our muscles, our brain, and our very life. The way we do this is by the metabolism of food. To better understand the energy production process in your own body, and to fully understand *why* you need to eat, it helps to visualize an electrical power plant that uses coal to produce electricity. As humans, we use food instead of coal, but the output—energy—is the same. Without coal, a power plant produces no electricity and is useless; without food, your body produces no energy for the cells in your body, and when that happens, you die. To help you fully understand your digestive tract and the process of digestion, the following section will detail what happens when food travels through your body.

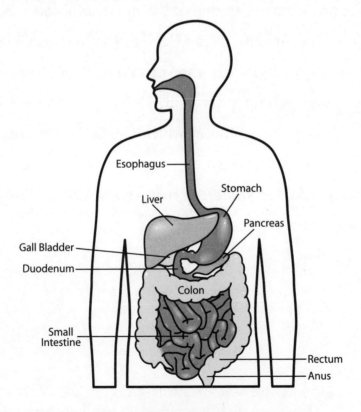

The Digestive System

Digesting Food

Is there anyone who can resist the smell and taste of fresh apple pie? In fact, how that yummy piece of apple pie travels down your digestive tract highway can serve as a perfect illustration of just how amazing—and complex—the journey from food to energy in the human body truly is.

Digestion of food, which leads to the production of energy, actually begins in the mouth. Yes, that's right—you immediately begin to digest your piece of apple pie the moment it goes from fork to mouth. In the mouth there are a number of structures that begin the digestion of food, starting with your teeth, the first thing that the piece of pie comes into contact with. Your teeth (original or not!) grind the pie into small, tiny pieces so that your tongue (a muscular organ that also allows you to taste your food via taste buds) can push the food down into the next part of the digestive system. However, before this takes place, the pie has already begun to be chemically broken down and digested by saliva, a watery secretion that's produced by salivary glands. Saliva not only lubricates food so that it passes easily through the rest of the digestive tract, but it also begins to chemically break down food so that it can be used for energy later down the tract.

So now that our piece of pie has been chewed up and lubricated, it can be swallowed and pass into the next part of the digestive tract, the pharynx and esophagus.

The pharynx (more commonly known as your throat) is a structure shaped like a funnel that connects the mouth to the esophagus, a long, muscular structure that goes all the way down to the stomach. During its trip down the esophagus, your apple pie is literally pushed down to the stomach by muscular contractions of the esophagus known as peristalsis.

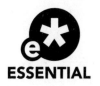

ESSENTIAL

It's worth noting that it's because of the peristalsis contractions that astronauts are able to eat and survive in space. If movement of food just depended on gravity, it would not only be impossible to digest food in a gravity-free environment, it would also be quite messy!

Once your pie hits the next organ of the digestive system—the stomach—things begin to get even more interesting. It's also important to know, for reasons that will become clear in the next section, that at the end of the esophagus where it meets the stomach is a ring of muscle called the cardiac sphincter, which literally closes off the end of the esophagus to keep the contents of the stomach from going back up into the esophagus.

In the stomach—which is about the size of two fists placed up against each other—food is essentially mixed and ground up both through muscular action and chemical reactions. The stomach secretes powerful enzymes and acids that break down your pie—now turned liquid—before it's passed to the small intestine, the real workhorse of the digestive system. The small intestine is around 10' long and made up of three segments called the duodenum, jejunum, and ileum. It's here in the small intestine where food is broken down even further with help from enzymes secreted into the small intestine by the pancreas and bile from the liver. After the proteins, carbohydrates, and fats in your apple pie liquid are broken down into small enough particles, they are absorbed through the walls of the small intestine and transported to the cells in your body, where organelles called mitochondria turn this food-fuel into energy.

FACT

Mitochondria are the tiny organelles in your cells that create the energy your body needs. They have their own DNA, which comes exclusively from your mother, unlike all other DNA which is from both your father and mother. The amount of mitochondria in your body's cells varies greatly. Some cells in the body can have thousands of mitochondria while others may have few to none. For example, muscle cells need large amounts of energy, so they can have upward of 2,000 mitochondria. Conversely, red blood cells have very few to no mitochondria.

Any food that's not usable as energy is passed further down the digestive tract into the large intestine, where water is removed from any remains of your piece of apple pie. Then whatever is left passes out of the body through the rectum and anus. Quite an incredible journey for one piece of apple pie, isn't it?

Just What Is Acid Reflux?

As you can imagine, on such a long and winding trip down the digestive highways, there are many potential potholes and obstacles that your piece of apple pie may have to overcome before it becomes part of the fuel that fires your human furnace. From simply not chewing your pie enough and having trouble swallowing (or, in the worst-case scenario, choking on it) to complex problems in anatomy or the biochemistry of digestion, the process of food to fuel isn't as simple as it might seem. One of the most common of these problems is when the digestion of food in the stomach—via secretion of digestive acids—doesn't work as seamlessly as it should.

ALERT

The latest data shows that acid reflux affects at least 10–20 percent of the population in the United States, and that number is going up. Acid reflux is the most common gastrointestinal complaint when patients visit their physicians, and it accounts for at least 4 percent of all visits to family practice physicians.

Remember back when we were talking about how food goes from the esophagus to the stomach? There's a valve of muscle at the juncture of the stomach and esophagus called the lower esophageal, or cardiac, sphincter, which keeps the contents of the stomach from going back up into the esophagus. When there's a problem with this mechanism—when the cardiac sphincter doesn't close all the way or opens too often—acid in the stomach, which is supposed to be there to help digest your food, can get into the esophagus. When this happens, the medical community calls it acid reflux or gastroesophageal reflux disease (GERD). While a little acid changing location may sound like no big deal, acid reflux is actually a huge deal in terms of your health.

Acid Reflux Symptoms and Warning Signs

"I get heartburn sometimes after I eat a spicy meal," some of you might be saying. "Does that mean I have acid reflux?" The answer to that question is . . .

maybe. If you're having the following symptoms at least twice a week, then it's worth getting an appointment with your doctor to discuss whether or not you do indeed have acid reflux.

While most people know the discomfort of acid reflux, such as constant burping, nausea after eating, uncomfortable stomach fullness and bloating, as well as the classic burning pain that moves from your stomach up into your throat, there are other signs of GERD that many people dismiss. Other symptoms of acid reflux include:

- **Acid regurgitation**—when the acid in the stomach comes all the way up into your throat, you may get a bitter, burning feeling in your mouth and throat. For people with acid reflux, this is very common in the early morning after eating a meal and late at night.
- **Extra saliva**—when your body senses something in your throat and mouth that shouldn't be there—in this case, acid—it causes you to make more saliva to wash out that offending agent. This sign is highly suggestive of acid reflux, yet is often dismissed by many people.
- **Sore throat**—who doesn't get a sore throat every now and then, right? However, it might very well be a sign of acid reflux. If you only develop a sore throat after meals, especially if you don't have other signs of an upper respiratory infection like a runny nose and fever, then you very well may be showing a sign of acid reflux.
- **Hoarseness**—as we grow older, our voice can change and many people take no note of it. Yet it may be caused by acid irritation of the vocal cords from an undiagnosed case of acid reflux. If you notice that your voice is growing more husky and hoarse for no apparent reason, let your doctor know.
- **Chest pain**—we're all taught that chest pain is a classic sign of having a heart attack, but it may also be a sign of severe acid reflux. Acid in the esophagus can elicit significant pain, so never ignore chest pain, especially if it gets worse when you exert yourself or exercise.
- **Coughing**—This one can fool a lot of people, but coughing can be the first presenting sign of acid reflux. Acid reflux can trigger a coughing spell that people will often attribute to allergies or some other nongastrointestinal cause, which then can significantly delay the diagnosis of acid reflux.

QUESTION

Why don't I get pain in my stomach from acid reflux?
The stomach is an amazing organ. It is an integral part in digesting all the food you eat by secreting acid from certain cells that break down the food so that nutrients can be absorbed in the intestines. Yet the cells that line the stomach are impervious to the acidity that bathes them, unlike the cells in the esophagus, which can be severely harmed by that same acid.

How Some People Develop Acid Reflux

It's worth noting that some reflux is normal as you age, and if it only happens once in a blue moon, then there's no problem. The problem lies when reflux happens on a daily—or more—basis. The question as to why it happens to some people and not others is still unanswered, but we do know that certain things can predispose you to developing acid reflux, such as:

- **Hiatal hernia.** This is a common cause of acid reflux, and while these hernias are more common as people get older, they can occur at any age. A hiatal hernia happens when the upper part of your stomach and the cardiac sphincter actually move up into the esophagus, making the valve between your stomach and esophagus leaky, which allows stomach acid to go back up, causing acid reflux.
- **Pregnancy.** Being pregnant, while generally a wonderful time in a woman's life, can also lead to acid reflux. It's caused by both the action of hormones as well as the physical pressure of the fetus growing in the uterus. Fortunately, symptoms generally subside after the baby is born.
- **Smoking.** While known to cause cancer and heart disease, smoking also increases your risk of developing acid reflux by potentially decreasing the amount of saliva produced, reducing the functioning of the cardiac sphincter, and increasing acid secretion.
- **Foods/late-night eating.** Eating right before bedtime, or eating some of the following foods, can definitely increase your chance of developing acid reflux. While not all the listed foods cause acid reflux in all people, the following are known to be common triggers:

- Alcohol
- Fried foods
- Fatty foods
- Chocolate
- Coffee/tea
- Acidic foods such as tomatoes
- Onions
- Spicy foods
- **Being overweight.** Being overweight, while contributing to many other disease processes such as diabetes, heart disease, and musculoskeletal problems, can also predispose you to developing acid reflux.

How Is Acid Reflux Diagnosed?

Unlike, say, strep throat, where a simple test can usually give a definitive answer on whether or not you have the infection, diagnosing acid reflux can be nebulous at best. Oftentimes, physicians treat it empirically—that is, they'll talk to the patient about lifestyle changes (i.e, not eating late at night, avoiding foods that seem to trigger the reflux, etc.), and also treat the symptoms like heartburn and stomach pain with prescription medications to see if the symptoms go away in 2–4 weeks and don't return. If so, great. If not, then physicians can move on to the following tests:

- **Upper endoscopy**—this is a procedure, usually done at an outpatient center, where a physician uses an endoscope—a small, finger-sized tube approximately 2–3' long with a light and camera on one end—to see the inside of a person's throat, esophagus, and stomach. While this might sound somewhat unpleasant, it actually is quite simple. Generally, a liquid anesthetic is sprayed in the back of the patient's throat to get rid of the strange sensation of the endoscope being placed there as well as to numb the patient's gag reflex. The physician will then carefully guide the endoscope down the patient's throat into the esophagus and stomach, all the while looking to see if there are any abnormalities. If so, the physician can do a biopsy—taking a small piece of tissue from either the esophagus or stomach—to send to a pathologist to see if there's any sign of inflammation or, in the worst-case scenario, cancer.

- **Esophageal manometry**—this is a test that tells your physician how well your esophagus is working in terms of its peristaltic actions (the rhythmic contractions of the esophagus as it pushes food down to the stomach) as well as how well the cardiac sphincter is working at closing and opening. Like the upper endoscopy, it also involves placing a thin tube, with sensors to measure muscle activity, down your throat and into your esophagus and stomach.

- **Barium swallow (esophagram)**—while this test was commonly done twenty or more years ago, it's being replaced by endoscopy. However, it's still utilized, so it's worth understanding. In this test, you swallow liquid barium and x-rays will be taken as the fluid goes down your esophagus into your stomach, allowing the physician to check for esophageal narrowing, scarring from stomach acid exposure, or hiatal hernia.

- **Esophageal pH monitoring**—this is considered by many gastroenterologists (physicians who specialize in disorders of the digestive system) to be the most accurate test in terms of measuring abnormal acid levels in the esophagus, the hallmark of acid reflux. This test can be used to check patients who fail empirical therapy and to monitor patients who are taking medications yet are still reporting symptoms. As in the upper endoscopy and esophageal manometry tests, the esophageal monitoring generally involves passing a small tube with a pH-monitoring probe at the end of it. This tube is then left in place for 24 hours, allowing the physician to accurately gauge how much acid is being passed up into the esophagus from the stomach.

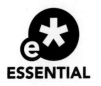

ESSENTIAL

Indeed, esophageal pH monitoring doesn't sound like much fun—and you probably don't want to walk around with a tube down your esophagus all day! Fortunately, you might not have to—there's now a wireless capsule that can be placed at the juncture of the esophagus and stomach, allowing your doctor to monitor the acid secretion without having a tube down your throat all day.

Complications and Dangers of Untreated Acid Reflux

It's true that everyone gets heartburn now and then. But the problem—a potentially life-threatening problem—occurs when heartburn happens on a regular basis and nothing is done about it. There can be multiple complications from ignoring your symptoms and hoping things will get better on their own, including:

- **Teeth problems**—untreated acid reflux can cause an increase in dental visits and dental bills. When acid comes back up from the stomach, not only does it cause problems in the esophagus, but when it reaches your mouth, it can cause destruction of the enamel of your teeth, leading to premature dental decay.
- **Voice and breathing problems**—as you can imagine, having your vocal cords bathed in acid over a long period of time will do nothing for a budding singing career, or even having a pleasant-sounding voice. In addition, people with untreated acid reflux can actually inhale the acid, which can cause multiple problems from difficulty breathing and shortness of breath to worsening of asthma.
- **Esophagitis**—left untreated, the acid from chronic reflux will damage the inner lining of the esophagus, causing chemical burns that can lead to inflammation, ulcers, and bleeding.
- **Esophageal stricture**—the chronic inflammation of esophagitis can cause an actual narrowing of the esophagus that's called a stricture. This narrowing can cause significant problems, from painful swallowing to actual choking, since there's very little room for your food to pass through.
- **Barrett's esophagus**—this is a condition where the cells that are normally found in the esophagus are literally changed from years of being assaulted by stomach acid to cells that are abnormal—that is, cells that can turn cancerous.
- **Esophageal cancer**—the most deadly result of untreated acid reflux is esophageal cancer. The rates of this devastating form of cancer have been steadily increasing, especially among African-American men. Esophageal cancer is divided into two main types: squamous cell car-

cinoma, which can affect any part of the esophagus, and adenocarcinoma, which generally develops in the lower part of the esophagus. Both types often cause no symptoms at first. It's only when patients start developing problems such as difficulty swallowing and unexplained weight loss that they go see their doctor, and by then, oftentimes the cancer has spread and it's too late to do anything.

FACT

The medical field just loves acronyms. Unfortunately they can be downright confusing, so it's useful to go over a few of them, especially since they all can cover acid reflux. *GERD* and *GORD* stand for gastroesophageal reflux disease. *FD* stands for functional dyspepsia.

By now, you should be convinced that acid reflux is a serious disease. Fortunately, there are multiple ways—in terms of behavioral changes, prescription medications, surgery, and even holistic therapies—that can not only treat acid reflux, but also prevent it from ever happening in the first place.

CHAPTER 2

Dietary Interventions for Acid Reflux

Now that you've gone down the digestive road, so to speak, it's time to talk about how you can change and modify what you eat and drink in order to minimize the chances of developing acid reflux. What goes into the digestive system has a profound effect on whether acid reflux occurs or not, and there are even some studies showing that a sensitivity to gluten may be underlying many cases of reflux.

Food and Acid Reflux

The food options that we have in the Western world today are truly mind-boggling. We literally have access to food 24 hours a day, 7 days a week, in an abundance that would have made a decadent Roman emperor blush. Blueberries from Chile, sushi from Japan, fish from the Arctic Ocean—what most of us can have to eat is really just a matter of what we want and how much we want to pay for it. But when it comes to food for those who suffer from acid reflux, the list of foods can shrink considerably, and for some people, may seem downright draconian.

ESSENTIAL

Historically there are varied food remedies for acid reflux. Ancient midwives in several cultures would give ginger, coriander, and cilantro for patients to chew on to relieve symptoms. The Malawi tribe in Africa boiled the root of the jasmine plant to help with heartburn.

Yet what foods seem to trigger acid reflux is an ever-evolving list. Ask one patient and he'll say, tomatoes and garlic are the culprits. Yet ask another patient and he'll tell you just the opposite—that tomatoes and garlic are just fine—it's grapes, broccoli, and yogurt that trigger his acid reflux.

But don't fret—there are some good studies showing that, for most people, certain foods seem to help soothe the discomfort of acid reflux while others seem to fan the flames. As you read on you'll learn about the foods you might want to avoid as well as some foods that may be useful in calming your acid reflux.

Beverages

It's not just food of course that's put down your esophagus—the beverages you drink can also have a profound effect on whether or not acid reflux develops. And one of those drinks might be one of the most widely consumed beverages in the world: coffee.

Coffee

Can people with acid reflux still enjoy a morning cup or two of java without feeling guilty about it? The answer to that isn't as easy as a yes or no. It is known that coffee induces lowering of the cardiac sphincter pressure, meaning that there's a greater chance for acid to come back into the esophagus from the stomach. Coffee is also known to stimulate gastric acid secretion and slow gastric emptying, two more things that can contribute to acid reflux. Because of these things, many physicians recommend that patients with acid reflux avoid coffee, but in reality, there's no consistent studies showing that coffee does actually promote reflux. Therefore, the best advice for patients with reflux is to stop their coffee consumption for at least a week to see if there's any improvement in their symptoms. If so, then it's probably time to put away your favorite coffee cup; however, if there's no improvement, then feel free to have that jolt of caffeine in the morning, knowing that you're not doing yourself any harm in the process.

Alcohol

As in the case of coffee, there's conflicting data on what role—if any—alcohol consumption plays in the development and exacerbation of acid reflux. A comprehensive review article in the *American Journal of Gastroenterology* discussed the many ways that alcohol consumption can contribute to both development and worsening of acid reflux, including reducing the cardiac sphincter pressure and increasing acid secretion in the stomach, as well as increasing gastric emptying, leading the authors of the study to conclude that "alcohol tends to facilitate or cause gastroesophageal reflux and esophageal mucosal damage, regardless of the type of alcoholic beverage involved." However, there are more recent studies showing no relationship between alcohol consumption and reflux. In a case-control study out of Norway, researchers compared 3,153 patients who had acid reflux with 40,210 without reflux symptoms. After looking at various factors that correlated various lifestyle factors such as smoking and alcohol use, the authors of the study concluded, "Alcohol, coffee, and tea do not seem to be risk factors for reflux." So again, the best course might be to forgo your glass of wine or bottle of beer at night for a week to see what happens with your reflux symptoms and change—or not—your lifestyle accordingly.

ESSENTIAL

Who doesn't like to have some cookies and milk or a bowl of ice cream before bed? Well, people with acid reflux should definitely not partake of this tradition. Eating at night for those with reflux can cause many problems, since often the food eaten is food that can exacerbate reflux. Second, by lying down to sleep you decrease pressure on your lower esophageal sphincter and if there's food in your stomach, it makes it easier for the acid that is trying to digest your nighttime snack to rise back into your esophagus.

Soda/Pop

Most people will tell you to stay away from pop and other carbonated beverages if you have acid reflux. Perhaps they're basing their advice on studies like one published in 2006 in the *Journal of Gastrointestinal Surgery*. In this study, researchers performed manometry studies on nine volunteers after they drank either tap water or carbonated beverages. Tap water, as might be expected, caused no changes in cardiac sphincter tone. Carbonated beverages, on the other hand, decreased the strength of the lower esophageal sphincter. Of course, like studies on coffee and alcohol, there is other data that shows that drinking soda and other carbonated beverages has no effect on acid reflux. In a 2010 review article, the authors examined multiple studies on the relationship between soda and other carbonated beverages on acid reflux and concluded that "based on the currently available literature, it appears that there is no direct evidence that carbonated beverages promote or exacerbate GERD." So, while soda isn't the healthiest of beverage choices, having one now and then probably isn't going to hurt in regard to your acid reflux; but again, it is a good idea to give up soda for a week to determine whether it affects your reflux symptoms.

Food

Like the studies regarding beverages and acid reflux, there's a plethora of articles touting this diet or that food to either avoid or improve your acid reflux. Now, while it can be useful to read about the experience of others and see what works for them, you should always keep in mind what the actual research shows, as well as what works for you.

High-Fat Diet

There have been multiple reports that link acid reflux with a high-fat diet, and studies tend to bear that wisdom out. A 2005 report in the journal *Gut* (very appropriate, don't you think?) showed the results of a cross-sectional study of 371 men and women examining their dietary intake and the risk of GERD. The researchers used a standardized questionnaire (the Gastroesophageal Reflux Questionnaire) to follow several indices of acid reflux, including severity, frequency, and onset; in addition, they used what's known in research as the Block 98 Food Frequency Questionnaire to follow what type of foods were consumed. By analyzing data from these questionnaires, the researchers were able to determine that a high-fat diet caused acid reflux symptoms, while a high-fiber diet (more on that in the next section) correlated with a lower risk of GERD.

ESSENTIAL

Other high-fat foods that can cause acid reflux include: French fries, butter, cheese, high-fat cuts of red meat, deep-fried foods, sour cream, potato chips, cream sauces, ice cream, and whole milk among others.

The association between a high-fat diet and acid reflux symptoms has been correlated in other studies. An early study in 1989 used 24-hour pH monitoring to look at the association between high-fat diets and reflux symptoms in patients with GERD. The researchers showed that those people with reflux had a higher acid exposure in their esophagus when compared to people without reflux. This study was correlated in a later study in which researchers again showed that in people with acid reflux, a high-fat diet induces longer acid exposure time in their esophagus, thereby exacerbating their reflux symptoms.

Fiber

Eating foods high in fiber can help with your acid reflux symptoms. Two food groups that fulfill that role—and have a lot of other beneficial effects in addition to helping with your acid reflux—are fruit and vegetables.

As discussed in Chapter 1, one of the most significant problems that can arise from untreated acid reflux is Barrett's esophagus, which is a definitive risk factor for esophageal cancer. The good news is that a diet high in fruit and vegetables—in addition to giving you the fiber you need to help your acid reflux—can also help reduce the risk of Barrett's esophagus and esophageal cancer. An article published in 2008 in the *American Journal of Gastro-enterology* discussed a case control study examining the effects of fruit and vegetables on the development of Barrett's esophagus. In this study of over 600 men and women with known acid reflux, the researchers showed that those men and women who had a diet high in fruit and vegetables had a statistically lower incidence of developing Barrett's esophagus when compared to those people whose diet was low in fruit and veggies. Another study published in 2013 echoed these results, showing that among 1,859 people, those who had a higher intake of dark green vegetables had a lower risk of developing Barrett's esophagus. This is good news because again, having Barrett's esophagus puts you at risk for developing cancer of the esophagus. But the even better news is that eating your fruit and veggies also protects you against esophageal cancer.

QUESTION

What exactly is fiber?
Fiber is the part of plant foods that is resistant to digestive enzymes and therefore not digested. There are two types of dietary fiber, soluble and insoluble. Soluble fiber slows digestion and helps your body absorb vital nutrients from foods. Soluble fiber retains water so it creates a gel used during digestion. Oat bran, barley, nuts, seeds, beans, lentils, peas, and some fruit and vegetables are sources of soluble fiber. Insoluble fiber helps speed food passing through the intestines and fosters bowel regularity. Wheat bran, vegetables, and whole grains are all sources of insoluble fiber.

Low-Carbohydrate/Glycemic-Index Foods

People have been using a low-carb/low-glycemic-index food diet for decades to combat obesity and all the associated health related problems the come with being overweight. There are studies that show that along with weight loss, a low-carb diet can actually decrease your acid reflux symptoms.

ESSENTIAL

Glycemic index is a measurement done on foods to see what their impact is on your blood sugar. High-glycemic-index foods, such as sodas and candy, cause your blood sugar levels to spike rapidly. Lower-glycemic-index foods, like apples, won't cause such a rapid spike. While nothing is absolute, it's highly accepted that low-glycemic-index foods are much healthier for you than high-glycemic-index foods, and a list of both can be found on a ny reputable medical site online.

One of the first studies to show this was a case study of five patients showing that after starting a low-carb diet, their symptoms of acid reflux either significantly improved or totally went away. A later study done at the University of North Carolina looked at eight female patients aged twenty-three to fifty-four with a BMI ranging from 30–58 and all with symptoms of acid reflux. After just six days on a low-carb diet, all the study participants rated a significant decrease in their acid reflux symptoms including nausea, bloating, and a burning sensation in the esophagus and throat. In addition, the researchers also conducted a 24-hour pH monitoring on each of the participants and found that the low-carb diet significantly decreased the amount of acid being secreted into the esophagus. With preliminary studies like these, it might be worth trying out a low-carb/low-glycemic-index diet to help in both losing weight and improving acid reflux.

Gluten-Free Eating and Acid Reflux

Gluten is a generic term used to describe proteins in certain grains, namely wheat, barley, and rye. It is not present in other grains such as rice, maize, millet, or corn. Gluten intolerance is a disease in which people who eat foods that contain wheat, barley, or rye (or even other nongluten grains that have been processed with these gluten-containing grains) can develop a number of both gastrointestinal and nongastrointestinal symptoms ranging from diarrhea and weight loss to more complex issues such as fatigue, depression, and other neurological symptoms.

FACT

Gluten sensitivity has been increasing in prevalence and is thought to affect millions of people around the world, although it is more commonly found in female Caucasians. For reasons scientists aren't sure of yet, people with gluten sensitivity have significant reaction in their gastrointestinal tract to gluten, leading to the previously mentioned symptoms.

Until recently most researchers worked on the assumption that people with gluten sensitivity only had health issues pertaining to interactions of the gluten protein in the small bowel. However, more and more studies have been released showing that not only can gluten and gluten sensitivity negatively impact the small bowel, but there may also be a significant connection between gluten and acid reflux. An example of one such study was published in the journal *Diseases of the Esophagus*, which discussed the fact that up to 60 percent of patients with untreated gluten sensitivity have symptoms such as acid reflux and other problems of the upper gastrointestinal tract.

Since getting someone with gluten sensitivity on a gluten-free diet can significantly reduce—and sometimes completely get rid of—all their classic symptoms such as stomach discomfort and diarrhea, it stands to reason that going gluten-free could also significantly help people whose acid reflux symptoms are triggered by gluten, and there are now studies backing up that hypothesis. One of the first studies, published in the journal *Gut*, did a retrospective study on 205 male and female patients aged eighteen to sixty-six years with celiac disease, along with 400 male and female patients who didn't have problems with gluten. The researchers showed that not only did patients with gluten sensitivity have a higher rate of reflux when compared to those patients without the sensitivity, but that putting gluten sensitive patients on a gluten-free diet significantly decreased all their symptoms, including acid reflux. This led the authors to conclude that "a gluten-free diet significantly decreased the relapse rate of GORD [gastroesophageal reflux disease] symptoms."

Another more recent study examined the effects of a gluten-free diet in patients with reflux in an even more detailed manner. In this study, researchers examined 105 patients with celiac disease, 29 of whom had reflux symptoms. Over a two-year study, the researchers showed that in those patients who had reflux symptoms, putting them on a gluten-free diet resolved their symptoms in 86.2 percent of the cases. What's even more exciting is that after six months, 80 percent of those on a gluten-free diet continued to be symptom-free, even without taking any prescription medications like PPIs (proton pump inhibitors, the mainstay pharmacological treatment of reflux). This led the authors to conclude that "a GFD [gluten-free diet] could be a useful approach in reducing GERD symptoms and in the prevention of recurrence. Furthermore, the present findings suggest that nonpharmacological treatment could be a useful alternative for many adult CD [celiac disease] patients with NERD [nonerosive reflux disease]."

Finally, another study published in 2011 again looked at the relationship of gluten sensitivity and reflux and the usefulness of a gluten-free diet in decreasing reflux symptoms. In this study, 133 gluten sensitive patients were matched with 70 control patients (those without gluten sensitivity). Out of those initial 133 gluten-sensitive patients, 53 of them completed symptom questionnaires every three months for the first year of the study, and then approximately four years after their diagnosis. The results of the study again confirmed that there is significant evidence pointing to a relationship between gluten sensitivity and acid reflux: There was a significantly higher percentage of patients with gluten sensitivity reporting acid reflux symptoms when compared to control patients without gluten sensitivity. In addition, after only three months on a gluten-free diet, patients had a rapid resolution of their reflux symptoms, leading the authors to conclude that "GERD symptoms are common in classically symptomatic untreated CD patients.

The GFD [gluten-free diet] is associated with a rapid and persistent improvement in reflux symptoms that resembles the healthy population."

So with all this evidence, can we conclusively say that everyone with acid reflux has gluten sensitivity? No, we can't. However, it might be wise if you have acid reflux to talk to your doctor about getting tested for gluten sensitivity, or, even easier, feel free to put yourself on a gluten-free diet for at least two months to see if your symptoms significantly improve. If they do, not only have you saved yourself a trip to your doctor, but you've just made your life a whole lot healthier and happier as well!

Creating Food Plans to Manage Symptoms

Preparing, cooking, and eating the right foods—meaning foods that don't precipitate or make your acid reflux worse—is one of the most basic things you can do to help prevent your acid reflux. While there are some great recipes in this book that can help you do just that, it's wise to remember some basic tips on how to create food plans that can help you not only manage but also prevent your acid reflux:

- **Cook lean.** Make sure the food you're preparing and cooking isn't fatty. Fat is a known trigger for acid reflux, so if it's not there in the first place you won't have to worry about it.
- **Try broiling, baking, or roasting food** rather than frying, which again can add unwanted fat to your diet.
- **Skip the hot sauce, cayenne pepper, and other spices that can exacerbate reflux.** Go instead for herbs like basil, thyme, and dill that can flavor your foods without triggering reflux.
- **Remember about portion control**—while it's commonly thought that bigger is better, in terms of food for people with acid reflux this old adage isn't correct. By eating smaller portions in a slow, mindful way, you'll not only have time to enjoy your food more, but you'll also be greatly lowering the chances that your food will cause acid reflux.

CHAPTER 3

Lifestyle Changes
for Acid Reflux

One of the great disservices Western medicine has imparted upon society is the notion that the mind and body are disconnected. The fact of the matter is that whatever goes on in your mind—your thoughts, your emotions—influences how the rest of your body works—or in the case of acid reflux, doesn't work properly. This chapter discusses some lifestyle changes that very well might help with your acid reflux symptoms, and your overall health in general.

Stress

In today's society, stress is at such a high rate that physicians can't seem to write prescriptions fast enough for antidepressant and antianxiety drugs, medications that can help mask the pain but do nothing for the underlying stress. Now, while some stress is good, it's chronic stress, or "dis-stress," that can lead to a number of illnesses and exacerbate others, including acid reflux.

ESSENTIAL

Prolonged, frequent, or intense stress can weaken the body's ability to resist infection and increase the likelihood of developing diseases. It can lead to permanent health issues including ulcers, high blood pressure, kidney disease, arthritis, and even allergic reactions.

The Biology of Stress

The hypothalamic-pituitary-adrenal (HPA) axis plays a major role in the health of both your mind and body. This intricate connection between your brain and endocrine system exerts a wide influence over your health, and many researchers suggest that the HPA axis is being overtaxed by our stressful twenty-first-century lifestyles.

It all starts in the brain with the hypothalamus, a specialized glandular area of the brain that some consider the master gland, which acts as a controller of the pituitary gland. During times of stress—physical, emotional, or mental—the hypothalamus releases corticotropin-releasing factor (CRF), which in turn signals the pituitary gland to release adrenocorticotropic hormone, or ACTH. This hormone then travels through the bloodstream to the adrenals, two small, triangle-shaped glands that are located on the top of the kidneys. When ACTH reaches the adrenals, it causes them to release even more hormones that affect how your body and mind deal with stress, in either a positive or negative fashion.

FACT

There are a number of studies showing how stress can influence and worsen acid reflux. One of these, published in 2010 in Norway, was a population-based study of over 65,000 men and women examining the relationships between stress and symptoms of acid reflux. The researchers were able to conclude that common, everyday stressors such as "high job demands, low job control, job strain, low job satis-faction, time pressure and self pressure were positively associated with the risk of GERD symptoms."

Reducing Stress

While it would be wonderful to have the financial means to live a stress-free life, the vast majority of us simply aren't ever going to be able to live that life. But don't worry; there are ways—besides running off to Tahiti!—that can help you reduce the stress in your life and therefore improve your over-all health as well as reduce your acid reflux symptoms.

One of the most widely studied and effective ways to reduce the burden of stress is through the study and practice of mindfulness. This stress reduc-tion method is based on learning how to achieve a certain level of con-sciousness that is best described as a nonjudgmental moment-to-moment awareness of one's own self both in terms of mind and body.

In terms of acid reflux, mindfulness-based stress reduction techniques as well as more traditional psychotherapy have also proved their worth via multiple studies. In a paper published in 2000 in the journal *Gastroenterol-ogy*, researchers examined 95 patients with functional dyspepsia—a com-mon gastric complaint that can include acid reflux—and looked at how psychotherapy could help. In this randomized, controlled trial, the authors of the paper showed that psychotherapy could decrease the symptoms of dyspepsia. A more recent paper published in 2013 confirmed these results, showing that even brief sessions of psychotherapy can be "a reliable method to improve gastrointestinal symptoms . . . in patients with functional dyspep-sia." In terms of mindfulness-based therapies, a paper published in 2014 per-formed a meta-analysis on a number of other studies and concluded that "studies suggest that mindfulness based interventions may provide benefit in functional gastrointestinal disorders."

If you'd like to explore the benefits of mindfulness, a good place to start trying mindfulness in your daily routine can be found at the University of California Los Angeles Mindfulness Research Center website (*www.marc .ucla.edu*). Here, you'll find a number of free, guided meditations that will help you start to become more mindful.

Smoking Cessation

The number of former smokers in the United States now outnumbers the number of current smokers, and that's a statistic we all should be happy about. There's a plethora of data showing that not only does smoking greatly increase your risk for killers such as heart disease and cancer, but it can also play a significant—and problematic—part in acid reflux.

One of the earliest studies to postulate how smoking is involved in the pathogenesis of acid reflux was published way back in the pre-Internet era in 1990 in the journal *Gut*. In this study, researchers looked at a group of twenty-six smokers, aged thirty-three to sixty-three, and performed various tests on them, including manometry and esophageal pH monitoring. The researchers found that cigarette smoking directly caused both lowering of the cardiac sphincter pressure and an increase in acid secretion, leading the authors to conclude that "cigarette smoking probably exacerbates reflux disease by directly provoking acid reflux and perhaps by long lasting reduction in lower esophageal sphincter pressure."

There are plenty more studies that back up the idea that smoking and acid reflux are associated. One in 2001 demonstrated that smoking increases the incidence of acid reflux via increasing acid in the esophagus, while another cross-sectional study of 2,680 Japanese men and women, published in 2011, reported that cigarette smoking was "significantly associated with overlaps among GERD, FD [functional dyspepsia], and IBS [irritable bowel syndrome] in Japanese adults."

While the studies linking cigarette use to acid reflux should be clear to even the most closed-minded cynic, there are even more reasons not to smoke. Besides being linked to acid reflux, smoking is also a causative factor in both Barrett's esophagus and esophageal carcinoma. A 2012 article examined data from five studies on cigarette smoking, Barrett's esophagus, and esophageal carcinoma. After analyzing all the data, the authors of the study confidently concluded that "cigarette smoking is a risk factor for BE [Barrett's esophagus]." In a prospective cohort study on 411 patients with Barrett's esophagus published in 2013, researchers showed that the risk of developing esophageal carcinoma was significantly increased by smoking cigarettes. From an even more recent study, published in 2014, researchers analyzed data from 24,068 men and women followed over a four-year period and again showed that smoking was associated with the development of both Barrett's esophagus and esophageal cancer.

Quitting Smoking

First off, there are a number of ways to replace the nicotine that is the major addictive component of tobacco. A number of NRTs (nicotine replacement therapies), originally only available with a doctor's prescription, can now be bought over the counter without a prescription and include nicotine gum, patches, and lozenges. While all are roughly equally effective, some people prefer the ease of using a patch once a day, while others, especially those smokers who enjoy the hand-to-mouth movement that smoking provides, will do better with the gum or lozenges (as having to put the gum or lozenges in your mouth multiple times a day crudely mimics the hand movements of smoking a cigarette). There's also a nicotine nasal inhaler to curb that cigarette craving, but you'll need a doctor's prescription for that. The bottom line for all these products is that they can help reduce the actual chemical addiction (of nicotine) that cigarette smoking causes and thus make it easier to quit smoking. None of them will, however, be a magic bullet, and unless you're ready to give up the smokes, don't make the erroneous conclusion that you can smoke *and* use NRTs at the same time—this is a sure-fire way to give yourself nicotine poisoning which can cause very unpleasant symptoms including a rapid heart rate, anxiety, and vomiting.

Besides NRTs, there are also non-NRT medications that are prescription only. Bupropion is a medication that was first developed to treat depression, but through a number of studies it was found that it also was effective in helping people quit smoking. It does this through raising the levels of a chemical called dopamine in the brain, something that nicotine also does.

It's thought that because of this, the urge for smokers to light up to raise dopamine levels is blunted, and hence, no urge to smoke.

The newest smoking cessation prescription medication, varenicline, goes one step further than bupropion in actually acting as a nicotine mimic and partially blocking the effects of nicotine in the brain. Both these medications seem to be effective in helping smokers give up the habit, but as in the case of NRTs, bupropion and varenicline are *not* magic bullets—if you're not ready to quit smoking, none of these smoking cessation aids will probably do you much good.

ESSENTIAL

While it may sound funny to nonsmokers, one of the hardest aspects of quitting smoking for some cigarette users is what to do with their hands. After 20, 30, even 40 years of putting a cigarette into your mouth multiple times a day, it's a habit that needs to be fed if people are to quit the smoking habit. And so, feed it—with carrots, celery sticks, or apple slices. It'll take the place of putting a cigarette in your mouth and be healthy for you to boot!

Finally, it's worth asking the following question—even if you do quit smoking, will it actually help relieve your acid reflux? Fortunately, the answer to that question is probably yes, an answer borne out by studies like the one published in 2013 in the *American Journal of Gastroenterology*. In this paper, researchers examined data from a study out of Norway that included 29,610 men and women. Examination of the data revealed that those smokers who quit, when compared to those who didn't, had significant relief from their acid reflux symptoms. This is just one more reason to give up cigarettes once and for all.

Weight Loss

One of the biggest health issues that can contribute to acid reflux is obesity. A study from 2005 in the *American Journal of Gastroenterology* examined 453 men and women in a cross-sectional study to determine the prevalence and risk factors for acid reflux in employees of the Veterans Administration.

The authors definitely concluded that, "overweight and obesity are strong independent risk factors of GERD symptoms and esophageal erosions." A detailed review article published in 2008 examined the evidence linking reflux to obesity, with the authors coming to the conclusion that "overall, epidemiological data show that maintaining a normal BMI may reduce the likelihood of developing GERD and its potential complications."

FACT

BMI, or body mass index, is a calculation based on weight and height to get a measure of your body fat. This is important because people with higher amounts of body fat tend to have a higher BMI, and this isn't good for your health. Having excess body fat is known to put you at higher risk for multiple diseases including cancer, diabetes, and stroke.

So if obesity can cause acid reflux, can losing weight decrease or even cure the symptoms? Fortunately, data seems to point to an answer of yes to that question. An early study published in 1999 examined the effects of weight loss on thirty-four obese men and women with reflux over a six-month period. After examining the data, the researchers found a "significant association between weight loss and improvement in symptoms of GORD," concluding that "patients who are overweight should be encouraged to lose weight as part of the first-line management." A more recent study, reported in 2013, looked at data from Norway among 29,610 men and women. As in the study from 1999, researchers again showed that obese patients with reflux who lost weight had a significant improvement in their symptoms. Finally, a prospective intervention study, also published in 2013, was even more encouraging regarding weight loss and acid reflux. Among those 332 overweight and obese men and women studied, those who lost the most weight at the end of the six-month study showed the most improvement in their acid reflux symptoms and in fact, the researchers determined that "a structured weight-loss program can lead to a complete resolution of GERD symptoms."

Methods for Losing Weight

Of course, when it comes to obesity, weight loss, and acid reflux, the question is "How do I lose weight?" While entire books have been written about this, and knowing that one weight-loss program doesn't work for everyone, there are some reasonable steps that can be taken by just about everybody who's committed to losing weight.

Mindfulness, besides being useful in managing stress, has been also shown in multiple studies to potentially help in both losing weight and maintaining weight loss. Authors of a 2013 review paper on mindfulness in the treatment of obesity and eating disorders concluded that "mindfulness approaches can improve or extend long-term health outcomes in persons with eating disorders and is also associated with a reduction in overall food consumption, healthier food choices, and practices that slow the eating process among the obese population."

Another method of weight loss is food portion control. There have been numerous studies done on food portioning and the burgeoning obesity epidemic, such as one published in 2005 in the *Journal of Nutrition*. After careful analysis, the authors of the study concluded that, "excessive food portions, particularly of energy-dense foods, contribute to the overconsumption of energy [and calories]. Telling people to simply 'eat less' is not likely to be an effective solution, because it is not just large portion sizes that increase energy intake, but rather large portions of energy-dense foods." Because of this and other studies like this, people looking to lose weight successfully should focus on the importance of not only being mindful of what foods they eat, but also the portions they eat. In addition they should increase their portions of foods that are high in nutritional value/less energy dense, such as fruit and vegetables.

Exercise

Be it in the gym or in your basement, exercise is another critical component of weight loss. Just about everyone knows that exercise is good for everything from losing weight to defeating health disease to improving your sexual health. But what you might not know is that there are studies showing that an increase in physical activity and exercise can help protect you against acid reflux. A 2004 paper in the journal *Gut* reported on a case-control study involving 3,153 men and women with acid reflux and compared them to 40,210 people without reflux. The authors of the study showed that just exercising (jogging, cross-country skiing, or swimming) 30 minutes a week decreased the risk of having acid reflux by 50 percent. A more recent study published in 2012 in the *World*

Journal of Gastroenterology reported on a cross-sectional survey done among 4,910 Swedish men and women aged forty to seventy-nine examining physical activity, obesity, and reflux. Like earlier studies, this one showed that "intermediate frequency of physical activity was associated with lower occurrence of GERD among individuals."

Dining Out

Many people are able to stick to their weight-loss routines at home but falter when it comes to dining out. So what are you supposed to do when you go out to eat? This is a great question. Many people are totally sincere in getting a handle on their obesity, yet feel that they can't go out with friends and family and not eat, or just order celery sticks and water. As in the case of obesity and weight loss, there are multiple books written on this one subject alone, but some basic tips when it comes to social gatherings and dining out are as follows:

- **Try to eat some low-calorie, nutritionally dense food** (such as fruit, veggies, and a handful of nuts) before you go out. That way you'll be less hungry—and therefore less tempted—to take advantage of the all-you-can-eat buffet.
- **Drink plenty of water.** While water itself won't fill you up and satisfy your hunger, it will put something in your stomach and make it less likely you'll overeat.
- **Order wisely.** Just because everyone else at the table is getting a 16-ounce porterhouse with mashed potatoes and gravy doesn't mean you have to. Fortunately, most restaurants now have on their menus what they call healthy choices. Take a look at those and choose wisely.
- **Feel free to say no!** It's okay and not rude to turn down the offer of a double-layered chocolate cake smothered in ice cream for dessert. Or for that matter, any other food that you know is going to break your diet-meal bank. It's your health, and if those you're dining with care at all about you, they'll understand.

CHAPTER 4

Medications

In today's world there is no shortage of pharmaceutical choices for pain relief. In fact it seems like every day there is a new "miracle" cure for acid reflux. But how do you sort though all the medication options and how do you know which one is best for your acid reflux? This chapter discusses the medication options available for acid reflux so you can make an educated decision about which route you may want to take. Remember, not every medication works the same for every person and you (with advice from your doctor) may have to try a few options before you find the perfect fit for your individual case.

Talking to Your Doctor

Pharmaceutical companies spend billions of dollars each year on advertising aimed directly at consumers (you) on top of the tens of billions they spend marketing to physicians. There is nothing wrong with patients asking their doctors questions about medications, and in fact many doctors encourage this. But when advertisements for the supposed latest and greatest (and probably most expensive) medications cause patients to demand their doctor give them these medications, it can cause a fracture in the doctor-patient relationship.

Medications for acid reflux and GERD are a prime example of meds advertised directly to consumers. Who hasn't seen the ad for "the little purple pill"? The best advice is, if you're curious or think that pill sounds just like what you need, ask your doctor about it. She'll likely tell you what she knows about it, what her thoughts are on it, and if it may help you. Doctors should not only offer their best advice to patients, but also act as someone who can help you cut through all the "questionable information" that can sometimes make medical decisions harder than they need to be.

In regard to acid reflux, what are the options for patients who, after losing weight, exercising, watching what they eat, and completing the other recommended lifestyle changes, are still having symptoms? Fortunately there are multiple pharmaceutical options out there for treating acid reflux.

Antacids

As discussed in Chapter 1, acid reflux causes pain and suffering when the acid in the stomach makes its way up into the esophagus. This acid in the esophagus can, and will, cause irritation of the esophageal lining, and in the process cause pain. So therefore, it sounds reasonable that one way to treat the symptoms of acid reflux would be to either stop the acid from coming up in the first place or, if you can't do that, at least do something to the acid so it doesn't cause irritation to the esophageal lining.

By taking this second route, antacids were born. Antacids are compounds that counteract acid in the esophagus, and therefore provide relief from acid reflux. The most common types are sodium or calcium bicarbonate and magnesium or aluminum hydroxide. Whatever the chemical composition, they all act quickly and effectively to neutralize acid in the esophagus, bringing quick relief to the symptoms of acid reflux.

FACT

There are many types and forms of antacids on the market—chewable tablets, liquid preparations, and even antacid gum. Studies comparing all three show that the antacid chewable gums provided the quickest and longest-lasting relief, with chewable tablets coming in second place, and liquids coming in last place.

While antacids are often a mainstay treatment for people with reflux, it's wise to remember that they're definitely not a cure. While antacids can help significantly and quickly decrease the pain and discomfort of reflux, they do nothing to stop the problem of acid escaping from the stomach into the esophagus. Their relief is also short-lived, meaning that for people with long-term reflux, antacids would have to be taken multiple times each day to provide adequate symptom relief. Antacids are not a curative therapy.

Alginate

Alginate is a polysaccharide, which is just a chemical name for a bunch of sugar molecules bonded together. Alginate occurs naturally in brown algae, but it's when alginate is combined with sodium or potassium bicarbonate that it can bring relief to sufferers of acid reflux. How it does this is actually pretty cool: When alginate and bicarbonate are combined, they interact with gastric acid in the stomach and form a foamy, chemical barrier that acts like a raft on water and literally floats on top of the acid. This foamy raft then can not only stop gastric acid from moving into the esophagus and causing acid reflux, but it can also move ahead of the acid as it floats on top of it and help protect the esophagus from damage.

Like antacids, alginate preparations can work very quickly at neutralizing the acid in reflux and thus provide quick relief from symptoms. There are also some studies that alginate preparations—the most common being the commercial OTC medication Gaviscon—can act as well as prescription proton pump inhibitor medications (more on these later in this chapter) in providing a 24-hour window of relief of symptoms.

ESSENTIAL

One of the challenges women have to face when pregnant is acid reflux, especially common in the third trimester. While it's important to be judicious in the use of any medications during pregnancy in regard to fetal health, studies have shown that alginate agents can be safely given throughout the pregnancy and can be quite effective.

Histamine Type 2 Receptor Antagonists (H2 Blockers)

H2 blockers, developed in the 1970s, were the first big prescription medications for acid reflux to show better effectiveness at treating the disease than over-the-counter medications. H2 blockers work by blocking a biochemical in the body called histamine, which does many things, one of which is stimulate acid secretion in the stomach. So if you can decrease acid secretion, you can decrease the amount of acid entering the esophagus, and therefore, decrease acid reflux.

QUESTION

Can H2 blockers cause vitamin deficiencies?
There are studies that show that H2 blockers can cause vitamin B_{12} deficiency. Therefore it is recommended that if you are using H2 blockers for your acid reflux you should take a B-complex vitamin as well. In one study, outlined in a 2013 article in the *Journal of the American Medical Association*, researchers conducted a case control study of 25,956 patients in California and came to the conclusion that "previous and current gastric acid inhibitor [H2 blockers and PPIs] use was significantly associated with the presence of vitamin B_{12} deficiency."

While H2 blockers can provide quick (though not as quick as antacids and alginate preparations) and very effective relief of acid reflux, they're not the perfect medicine. Multiple studies have shown that people can develop a tolerance to H2 medications, meaning that after taking the medication for a while, it will lose its effectiveness. So, while H2 blockers are very effective medications at both treating and preventing acid reflux, they work best for reflux that just occurs every now and then and are probably not the best option for when reflux is a chronic or frequent problem.

Which H2 Blocker to Choose?

Going to your local pharmacy to pick out an H2 blocker to treat your reflux might seem like a frustrating exercise. There are a number of these medications on the market, so to help out here's a list with their chemical name, brand name, and dosage

- Cimetidine (Tagamet)—200–400 mg once or twice a day
- Ranitidine (Zantac)—75–150 mg once or twice a day
- Famotidine (Pepcid)—10–20 mg once or twice a day
- Nizatidine (Axid)—150 mg twice daily (this one is only available through prescription)

Proton Pump Inhibitors (PPIs)

Proton pump inhibitors (PPIs) hit the acid reflux market in the 1990s and have continued in popularity since. They are by far some of the most widely prescribed medications on the planet and the most potent inhibitors of gastric acid secretion by the stomach. Without getting too complicated, they work by significantly inhibiting the proton pump in the stomach, which is the final common step of gastric acid secretion. PPIs work morning, noon, and night; they are the best medications on the market today for both stopping the symptoms of acid reflux as well as helping the esophagus heal from the damage caused by excess exposure to acid.

Studies have shown that PPIs work better than H2 blockers in both symptom relief and faster healing of the esophagus. Studies also show that, when compared to a placebo, PPIs at standard doses generally have a 30–35 percent efficacy for control of reflux. Of course, this means that there are a percentage of people who don't have resolution of symptoms; for these people, many physicians will recommend doubling the dose, although studies aren't clear as to whether this really helps give any more relief of symptoms.

While there are many advantages to PPIs, these meds do have their potential drawbacks, and some of them might be significant. The one potential drawback that has certainly gotten the most press—both in the medical community and with laypeople—is the risk of bone mineral density reduction and bone fractures. Because of the significant healthcare concerns this potential side effect raises, there have been numerous studies looking at this issue. A 2012 review article in the journal *Pharmacotherapy* reviewed fourteen studies on the potential association between PPIs, loss of bone mineral density, and fractures. Out of these fourteen observational studies, eight found an increased risk of hip fracture with the prolonged use of PPIs and five studies found an increased risk of spine fractures. Three studies examined the risk of bone mineral density loss and found no association with PPI use. The authors of this review article concluded that there is "a moderate increase in the risk of hip fracture and vertebral fracture associated with PPIs, although some studies showed conflicting results."

ALERT

There are studies—again, not conclusive—that associate PPI use with an increased risk of developing pneumonia and *Clostridium difficile*, both potentially life-threatening infections seen in hospitalized patients. This once again pounds the point home that prescription medications should only be taken if they're needed, and generally, for only the amount of time that they need to do their work.

However, don't let this information sway you into stopping your PPI, since again, the data still isn't crystal clear. A recent (2014) article in the journal *Current Treatment Options in Gastroenterology* looked at the most recent (at the time) data on the association between PPIs and bone fractures and came to the following conclusions: "There is a large body of observational evidence involving nearly 2 million participants that demonstrates there is an association between PPI therapy and risk of fracture. . . . The likely reason for this association is confounding factors and it is probable that PPI therapy is not a risk factor for fracture."

The bottom line is that there's some evidence that PPIs increase fracture risk, but it's far from conclusive. The best advice for those of you who take PPIs is to take them for as short a time as possible and if they're not working, even at higher doses, talk with your doctor about switching treatment plans.

Types of Proton Pump Inhibitors

Like H2 blockers, there are a number of proton pump inhibitors on the market today, and for good reason—they're effective, they're widely prescribed and used, and of course they make the pharmaceutical companies loads of money. So here's a list of the current ones on the market with their chemical name, brand name, and dosage. It also may help to know that, notwithstanding advertisements from pharmaceutical companies, there don't seem to be any major differences in the effectiveness of the medications in treating reflux (although to be fair, certain drugs work better in certain people than others).

- Esomeprazole (Nexium)—40 mg once daily
- Lansoprazole (Prevacid)—30 mg once daily
- Omeprazole (Prilosec)—20 mg once daily
- Pantoprazole (Protonix)—40 mg once daily
- Rabeprazole (Aciphex)—20 mg once daily

Prokinetic Medications

Besides the H2 blockers and PPIs—both of which are considered the mainstay of acid reflux treatment in terms of prescription medications—there are still other drugs recommended by physicians that fall into yet another category. Prokinetic drugs help the esophagus in its movements and thereby—in theory anyway—get rid of any excess gastric acid faster. This is "in theory" because studies have shown that prokinetic drugs only have a modest positive effect in decreasing the symptoms of acid reflux, and they can have some significant negative side effects. Because of this, these medications—including metoclopromide, domperidone, cisapride, and tegaserod—aren't (or shouldn't be) used routinely in treating acid reflux and should only be tried when H2 blockers and PPIs fail.

Future Medications

With even the best medications on the market—the H2 blockers and PPIs—providing no better than 30–40 percent effectiveness in patients, you can bet that pharmaceutical companies are scrambling to come up with more drugs to treat acid reflux that will work better and have fewer side effects.

One of the most promising types of medications that may very well be on the market in the not-too-distant future are drugs known as gamma-aminobutyric acid (GABA) type B receptor agonists. These medicines, currently in clinical trials, act by reducing both the lower esophageal sphincter relaxations and reflux events through their effect on the nervous system. In fact, the medical community already has one of these GABA type B receptor agonists available right now, a drug known as baclofen. In multiple trials, baclofen has been shown to significantly reduce acid reflux symptoms in patients; unfortunately, it also has a number of problematic side effects including dizziness, nausea, and vomiting that make it not particularly useful as a widespread medication in treating acid reflux. However, researchers are working on GABA receptor agonist drugs that maintain the favorable effects of baclofen without the negative side effects. One of these drugs, known as lesogaberan, has been shown in early studies to significantly decrease the lower esophageal sphincter tone and decrease reflux symptoms in a prompt and effective manner without the negative side effects of baclofen.

Besides the GABA type B receptor agonists, there are other medications in the pipeline that are showing promise in early clinical trials to treat acid reflux, including metabotropic glutamate receptor 5 antagonists, nitric oxide synthase inhibitors, and cannabinoid agonists. While some of these might pan out and others might fail in large clinical trials, the positive news is that science is marching on in the field of new medications for the treatment of acid reflux.

CHAPTER 5

Integrative and Holistic Therapies

The use of alternative and holistic therapies, both in the United States and around the world, is a major force in today's healthcare environment. Recent surveys show that around 40 percent of U.S. adults use some type of alternative therapy, and that number will most likely continue to increase. People want to have control of their own lives, and yet in modern mainstream medicine, that's one thing that's often taken away from them. By turning to treatments people can research and buy themselves, they can take back that control. In terms of acid reflux, the data regarding integrative and holistic therapies is few and far between. This chapter discusses the available information on alternative therapies for acid reflux and what shows some potential, and may be worthwhile to try.

Acupuncture

While it's true that acupuncture is used extensively to treat musculoskeletal problems, there's compelling data that suggests that this ancient form of Asian medicine can be useful in a variety of medical conditions, including acid reflux.

An intriguing study published in 2007 compared acupuncture to a PPI in providing relief for acid reflux. The patients in this randomized study were thirty men and women who had known acid reflux and were taking omeprazole (20 mg once daily) to control their acid reflux symptoms. They were then randomized into two groups: one taking 20 mg of omeprazole once daily along with acupuncture; and the other taking 20 mg of omeprazole twice daily. The results showed that those patients taking the PPI and receiving acupuncture had greater relief of their symptoms when compared to those patients taking the PPI twice a day, leading the authors to conclude that "adding acupuncture is more effective than doubling the proton pump inhibitor dose in controlling gastro-oesophageal reflux disease–related symptoms in patients who failed standard-dose proton pump inhibitors."

ESSENTIAL

You may need several weeks to months of acupuncture treatments to achieve your desired results. Consult with your acupuncturist on your treatment time frame, as you may need more frequent sessions initially if your symptoms are severe. Costs for acupuncture treatments can vary greatly, but some insurance companies may cover this procedure, especially if the acid reflux is causing a great deal of pain.

A more recent study published in 2010 further confirmed the usefulness of acupuncture in treating acid reflux. In this randomized six-week trial of sixty patients with confirmed acid reflux, researchers again showed that acupuncture was effective in inhibiting acid secretion (confirmed with 24-hour pH intraesophageal monitoring) and alleviating symptoms.

Hypnosis

Some people may think of hypnosis as a magician's trick or a hoax. The truth of the matter is that hypnosis is a very powerful technique that can induce powerful changes—both mental and physical—that modern-day science and medicine are just beginning to tap. An early study published in 1975 showed that hypnosis could decrease both gastric acid secretion and gut motility in female volunteers. In terms of acid reflux and other gastroenterological disorders, hypnosis has been shown in some early studies to be quite useful, as seen in a study from 2002 out of Britain. In this randomized, placebo-controlled study, 126 patients with functional dyspepsia (who have symptoms of acid reflux) were randomized to groups getting hypnosis, placebo and supportive therapy, or ranitidine at 150 mg twice daily. At the end of one year, those receiving hypnosis had a significant decrease in their symptoms such as pain and nausea, and in fact noted better symptom improvement than those taking the H2 blocker. If you are interested in exploring hypnotherapy you can go to the website of the National Board of Certified Hypnotherapists (*www.natboard.com*) to get a listing of hypnotherapists in your state.

Vitamins and Amino Acids

The sale of vitamins and other supplements is *big* business in the United States, as in billions of dollars of sales a year. There are quite a few supplements that show promise in helping prevent or treat a number of diseases, with some preliminary studies showing that some supplements help in treating reflux. A single-blind, randomized study published in 2006 examined the effects of a number of dietary supplements, including vitamins, amino acids, and melatonin, in the treatment of gastroesophageal reflux. Researchers in this study gave 351 male and female patients aged twenty-nine to fifty-nine either 20 mg daily of omeprazole or a dietary supplement that was composed of vitamin B_6, vitamin B_{12}, methionine, tryptophan, betaine, folic acid, and melatonin. At the end of the forty-day treatment period, 100 percent of those patients taking the supplement composition reported complete regression of their reflux symptoms, as compared to 67 percent of the patients taking the PPI who reported worsening of their symptoms.

Melatonin

Melatonin is often used to treat insomnia, with multiple studies showing its effectiveness. Research has also shown that melatonin may play a significant role in not only treating acid reflux, but also preventing it.

While melatonin is produced in the brain by the pineal gland and is intimately involved in the sleep/wake cycle of all mammals, it's also produced—at levels 400 times *above* that which is produced in the pineal gland—by cells in the human digestive system. We do know that melatonin plays an important role in protecting the digestive system—including the esophagus—from inflammation brought about by esophageal exposure to gastric acid. Because of this, studies are now being conducted looking at how supplemental melatonin can be used as therapy for acid reflux. In one such study published in the journal *Gastroenterology*, researchers studied thirty-six men and women with known acid reflux and put them into four study groups: one group that received no treatment, one group that received 3 mg of melatonin at night; one group that received 20 mg of omeprazole daily, and one group that received both omeprazole and melatonin. At the end of the eight-week study, those patients taking either melatonin alone or melatonin with omeprazole showed significant improvement in both their symptoms as well as in lower cardiac sphincter function, leading the authors to conclude that, "melatonin could be used in the treatment of GERD either alone or in combination with omeprazole."

Herbal Therapies for Acid Reflux

While herbal therapies are often derided by mainstream physicians as alternative or downright quackery, they couldn't be more wrong; a significant number of modern-day medicines that doctors write prescriptions for every day are derived from plant sources. Herbal therapies can be useful in a number of conditions including heart disease, cancer, and of course, acid reflux.

One herbal extract that shows promise is curcumin. This powerful substance has significant anti-inflammatory properties, making it a useful treatment for conditions in which inflammation plays a significant role (and as we in the scientific and medical communities are learning, chronic inflammation plays a role in most chronic diseases), including acid reflux. While human studies using curcumin in treating acid reflux are still in the preliminary stages, laboratory studies have shown that curcumin can cause a significant decrease of the inflammation of human epithelial cells brought about by high acid levels seen in reflux. A current research study is ongoing that will review and examine in detail any studies on curcumin pertaining to effect on multiple digestive disorders, including acid reflux.

ESSENTIAL

You may hear the terms *complementary*, *alternative*, and *integrative medicine* thrown about quite a bit, but what are they actually? First, they are modalities that aren't normally accepted as common or main-stream by physicians. Secondly, they are techniques and treatments that aren't generally taught to medical students (unless they take classes like mine on complementary and alternative medicine). Finally, they are therapies and treatments that aren't usually paid for by insurance companies.

Another plant-based therapy that can be useful in a variety of medical conditions—as well as making tasty candy—is licorice root. Early animal studies showed that both licorice root, as well as the chemical glycyrrhetinic acid, which is derived from the root, both act as potent anti-inflammatory agents in the rat gut. A 2010 study of glycyrrhetinic acid, again in rats, showed that it acted as both an anti-inflammatory agent and a potent reducer of gastric acid. Finally, a 2014 human study looked at the effects of a gum containing licorice extract on reflux symptoms. In this double-blind, placebo-controlled crossover trial, researchers studied twenty-four subjects with known acid reflux and had them chew either a placebo gum or the licorice extract gum after a meal that was known to exacerbate their reflux symptoms. Compared to those who chewed the placebo gum, subjects who chewed the licorice gum reported statistically significant decreases in acid reflux.

Another holiday favorite that may be of some benefit in helping sufferers of acid reflux is peppermint. While there are some Internet sites that warn patients with acid reflux to stay away from peppermint, published research shows the opposite. Peppermint has been shown to have positive effects on gastric emptying and cardiac sphincter pressure. Human studies have shown that the combination of peppermint and caraway oil is useful in alleviating the symptoms of functional dyspepsia, including acid reflux.

Finally, in terms of herbal therapies, one that holds promise in treating reflux and other digestive problems is artichoke leaf, which has been used in many traditional healing modalities for a variety of digestive disorders. A placebo-controlled, double-blind study published in 2003 examined the use of artichoke leaf extract on the symptoms of functional dyspepsia among 247 men and women. The researchers found that those patients taking the artichoke leaf extract had statistically significant improvement in many of their symptoms when compared to those taking a placebo.

D-Limonene

D-limonene is what makes up the major portion of citrus oils—from oranges, grapefruit, lime, and lemons. You've probably eaten it and not even known it, since d-limonene is used as a flavoring agent in such things as ice cream, sodas, baked goods, and juices.

Besides being a tasty food additive, d-limonene has many health-related activities. First it's great at dissolving gallstones. Studies show that it can be useful after gallstone surgery to dissolve those tiny stones that surgeons may miss. D-limonene also has anti-cancer activity, and early human studies have shown that it potentially may be useful for treating multiple cancers, including breast and colon cancers.

But while all that is good news, let's look at some data on how d-limonene can help with acid reflux. In one study on nineteen patients with chronic acid reflux, 1 gram daily of d-limonene caused complete resolution of symptoms in only two weeks. In another study, this one randomized, double-blinded, and placebo-controlled, thirteen patients with acid reflux were randomized to receive either 1 gram of d-limonene daily or placebo. As with the previously mentioned study, after two weeks 86 percent of the study participants had complete relief of their symptoms as compared to 29 percent that were taking the placebo.

Probiotics

Probiotics—or "good bacteria"—are found in certain foods like yogurt, kefir, and some hard cheeses. More and more studies are showing that taking probiotics—either in the foods you eat or as supplements—is vitally important in maintaining optimal health, and that includes the health of your digestive system.

ESSENTIAL

The study of probiotics is one of the hottest fields in medicine right now. There are new articles coming out literally every week in a variety of medical publications that show the vital importance of maintaining your intestinal flora for optimal health. Probiotics are so important that many doctors are now encouraging their patients to consume foods high in probiotics or to take a probiotic supplement.

While many people think that bacteria are bad (and yes, there are definitely certain types of bacteria that can make you sick), cutting-edge research is now showing otherwise. Science is now finally catching up to traditional societies in Eastern Europe and Russia who have known for centuries that eating fermented foods—foods high in probiotics—can help maintain a healthy digestive tract and fight off diseases. Just a small sampling of the most recent scientific literature yields a number of articles showing the importance of probiotics for everyone—men, women, young, and old. In fact, research has shown that as we age, the type of bacteria in our digestive system changes—not always for the better—and that these changes can be responsible for the maladies of the elderly, including acid reflux.

One way probiotics may be helpful for acid reflux—as well as for digestive health in general—is by controlling inflammation and increasing the health of the esophageal barrier, thus protecting against damage by stomach acid. While further research should shed more light on the many ways probiotics can help protect against acid reflux and other diseases, their use—as both a food and supplement—is something that many doctors heartily endorse for their patients.

CHAPTER 6

Surgery

Mainstream Western medicine has its flaws. However, there's no medical system, past or present, that can match the surgical methods and technology of twenty-first-century Western medicine. For example, laparoscopic surgical techniques have changed surgeries that in the past were dangerous and cost the patient a week in the hospital into safe, effective, out-patient surgeries. Because of advances like these, surgery for acid reflux is now a viable option for many more people than it used to be.

Should You Have Surgery?

Even with the advances in surgical methods surgery should not be considered right off the bat. You should be conservative when it comes to any invasive procedure. Surgery should be the last option, but an option nonetheless. So the question is what should prompt you to discuss getting surgery for acid reflux with your doctor? That's ultimately up to you and your doctor, but the following should be paramount in your consideration:

1. Is the acid reflux not controlled by the behavioral/preventive/pharmaceutical measures that have been discussed earlier in this book?
2. Are you having so many undesirable side effects from medications that you're not able to take them as you need to in order to control your acid reflux?
3. Are you having, despite the measures discussed earlier, further complications from your acid reflux such as ulcers, intractable pain, or the development of Barrett's esophagus?

If you're having any of these problems, you should consider at least having a sit-down with your doctor and surgeon to discuss what surgical options are available to you to see if they think it would be worth the risk.

If you and your doctor ultimately decide that surgery is the way to go, what should you expect next? First you'll have a pre-op, or preoperative, assessment and evaluation to determine if you're physically ready to go under the knife. This generally consists of a thorough evaluation to make sure acid reflux is what's truly causing your problems; a complete evaluation of your esophageal function; an assessment of any other factors that may come into play in the worsening of your acid reflux; and a complete physical, including EKG, to determine if you're healthy enough to have surgery.

Types of Surgeries for Acid Reflux

Surgery for acid reflux started becoming more popular and widespread back in the 1950s when a technique called fundoplication was perfected. During this surgery—which was initially performed by opening a rather large incision in your chest and abdominal area, but is generally now done laparoscopically—a surgeon visualizes the part of the esophagus that enters into the stomach. Then, she takes the top part of the stomach, wraps it around the lower end of the esophagus, and sutures, or sews, those parts together. The idea behind this surgical procedure is that by doing so, pressure will be increased at that area and thus help prevent acid from coming up from the stomach into the esophagus.

Of course, nothing is perfect, and fundoplication, while able to completely eliminate acid reflux symptoms when successful, isn't always successful. Failure rates—meaning patients continuing to have acid reflux—have been reported to be as low as 3 percent to as high as 20 percent. Yet recent studies have shown that fundoplication can be very effective in relieving acid reflux, even beating out PPIs. In one study on 63 patients with acid reflux, 90 percent of them reported complete elimination of their symptoms after six months. With results like these, fundoplication will continue to play an ever-evolving role in treating patients with recalcitrant reflux and GERD.

Bariatric Surgery

Bariatric surgery is generally a type of weight-loss surgery. As mentioned in Chapter 3, obesity is a significant risk factor for acid reflux, so it makes sense to postulate that major weight loss via bariatric surgery could help decrease the symptoms of reflux, and studies seem to bear that out. A review article published in 2009 looked at various modalities—lifestyle modifications, weight loss, dietary changes, and surgery—for improving acid reflux. The authors reported that, in terms of surgery, Roux-en-Y gastric bypass (RYGB) was the most effective in alleviating symptoms of acid reflux. This was in contrast to other types of surgery, in particular vertical banded gastroplasty (VBG), in which acid reflux symptoms remained the same or worsened.

FACT

There are many different types of surgery to treat obesity, with gastric bypass still being one of the most common and most effective. In Roux-en-Y gastric bypass, surgeons separate the smaller portion of the upper stomach from the lower stomach and reroute the small intestine; the net result is that the amount of food you can take in is considerably decreased.

Results of this study were confirmed in a more recent (2014) review article in the *Canadian Journal of Surgery*. As with results from a 2009 study, the authors found that Roux-en-Y gastric bypass (RYGB) was the most effective form of obesity surgery in decreasing or eliminating acid reflux. Their review showed that sleeve gastronomy tended to worsen acid reflux and gastric banding initially improved reflux symptoms, but that over time, some patients experienced recurring or worsening of symptoms. Based on their study, the authors concluded that "it appears that RYGB provides the best alleviation of symptoms associated with GERD and its comorbidities."

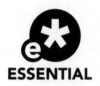

ESSENTIAL

While gastric bypass is still a common—and very successful—type of surgery for obesity, there are certainly others worth mentioning. Gastric banding—more commonly known as the Lap-Band—is a surgery where a band is placed around the upper stomach to decrease food intake. Vertical sleeve gastrectomy is a procedure in which a significant portion of the stomach is removed, leaving a tubelike structure. In gastric plication surgery, the stomach is folded inward and sutured into place, which again reduces the amount of food you can take in.

Electrical Stimulation for Acid Reflux

Modern technology has given physicians the ability to, in essence, shock the esophagus into behaving better and reducing acid reflux. The technique of using electrical stimulation to treat acid reflux, known more properly as LES-electrical stimulation therapy, is an exciting new avenue in treating acid reflux without having to resort to actual open-body surgery.

In LES-electrical stimulation therapy, physicians use an implantable electrical stimulator to provide electrical stimulation to the lower esophageal sphincter and, by doing so, increase the resting sphincter pressure and thereby decrease acid escaping from the stomach into the esophagus. A 2013 paper in the journal *Endoscopy* detailed the results of a twelve-month study of LES-electrical stimulation therapy in twenty-four men and women, aged forty-one to sixty-five, with acid reflux who were not getting acceptable relief of their reflux from medications, including PPIs. At the end of the study period (twelve months) 96 percent of patients were completely off their medications, leading the authors of the study to conclude that "LES-EST [electrical stimulation therapy] was safe and effective for the treatment of GERD." They found that there was "a significant and sustained improvement in GERD symptoms, reduction in esophageal acid exposure with elimination of daily PPI usage, and no stimulation-related adverse effects." If further studies are as positive as this one, I expect to see LES-EST being used much more frequently in the future to treat medication-resistant acid reflux.

FACT

In addition to using electrical stimulation, radio waves have also been used to help treat acid reflux. Radio-frequency (RF) induction is a technique in which doctors use a device to apply RF energy to the gastroesophageal junction to cause scarring that will, like other techniques, decrease the area in which acid can escape from the stomach and get into the esophagus. While short-term results are promising, long-term and larger studies are needed to see if this will be another tool in the fight against acid reflux.

Minimally Invasive Endoluminal Therapies

As you've seen throughout this book, there are a number of ways medical researchers have attempted to both prevent and cure acid reflux, from medications to surgeries to implanting electrical devices to shock the esophagus. Yet another technique in the medical toolbox is to implant certain inert substances into the distal esophagus, with the idea being that this can change the lower esophageal tone and thereby decrease acid reflux. While there have been over two decades of study on this approach, it's only been recently that polymer substances have been developed that have shown positive results in terms of safe implantation of the material, with very few procedure-related complications and short-term improvement of GERD symptoms. However, one of the injectable polymers with the brand name Enteryx was subjected to an FDA-mandated medical alert last year due to reports that erroneous injection of the polymer could cause serious complications, including death. Because of this the use of all polymers to treat acid reflux will most likely be put on the back burner until the situation can be resolved.

The Road to Recovery

Surgery—especially weight-loss surgery—can be a life-changing experience. But before you can go out and enjoy the new you, you're going to have to recover. First off, take it easy—your body has gone through some major stressors, so forget about hitting the gym for a while. You'll also have to eat differently due to the changes in your stomach from whatever surgery you've chosen. You'll need to eat smaller pieces of food, chew them longer, and drink plenty of fluids between meals. You also will need to talk to your doctor and nutritionist about taking supplements, because with certain surgical procedures you could be at risk of significant nutritional deficiencies without taking B-complex vitamins, including vitamin B_{12}, iron, calcium, and other vitamins and minerals. Remember that both weight-loss and acid reflux surgery isn't an end unto itself; if you go back to eating the wrong foods, drinking too much alcohol, and not listening to what your body is telling you, then despite the effort, cost, and pain involved in surgery, the chances of long-term success will be slim. Finally, the bottom line in any surgery—acid reflux, weight loss, or otherwise—is to know and discuss the risks and benefits with your surgeon, to be truthful to yourself about your expectations, and to be ready if the surgery doesn't go exactly as planned.

CHAPTER 7

Breakfast

Herbed Vegetable Omelet

This omelet is a simple way to add an extra serving of vegetables to your day.

INGREDIENTS | SERVES 2

Nonstick cooking spray, as needed
2 cups sliced white mushrooms
3 tablespoons low-fat milk
2 tablespoons sour cream
Salt and ground black pepper, to taste
2 tablespoons chopped green onions
1 tablespoon chopped chives
¼ teaspoon dried tarragon
4 egg whites
2 large eggs

Low-Fat Alternative

Fresh herbs and mushrooms give this omelet tons of earthy flavor. In the summer, use fresh herbs from your own garden. To cut back on saturated fat, try using 6 egg whites and passing on the yolks.

1. Heat a large skillet over medium-high heat and coat with cooking spray. Add mushrooms and cook until soft and liquid evaporates. Set aside.

2. In a small bowl, mix together 1 tablespoon milk, sour cream, salt, and pepper. Whisk well and set aside.

3. In a large bowl, mix remaining 2 tablespoons milk, green onion, chives, tarragon, egg whites, and eggs in a bowl; stir well.

4. Pour egg mixture into a large greased skillet over medium-high heat and let spread evenly over pan. Once center is cooked, cover egg with mushrooms. Loosen omelet with spatula and fold over.

5. Place omelet on a plate to serve and top with sour cream mixture.

Irish Oatmeal and Poached Fruit

This recipe will keep you going for hours! It has the perfect combination of slow-release starch and get 'em going fruit. The nuts will stave off hunger, too.

INGREDIENTS | SERVES 4

1 medium peach, chopped

½ cup raisins

1 tart medium apple, cored and chopped

½ cup water

3 tablespoons honey

½ teaspoon salt

2 cups gluten-free Irish or Scottish oats

1½ cups nonfat milk

1½ cups plain low-fat yogurt

1 cup toasted walnuts

1. In a medium saucepan, mix peach, raisins, and apple with water, honey, and salt. Bring to a boil and then remove from heat.

2. Mix oats and milk with low-fat yogurt in another medium saucepan. Cook according to package directions.

3. Add fruit to oatmeal and cook for 2–3 minutes on medium heat. Serve hot, sprinkled with walnuts.

Instant Oatmeal

Avoid instant oatmeal for breakfast, for cookies, and for making snacks. The oats in instant oatmeal are cut very thinly, and particle size is important to a low-GI food plan. The larger the particles, the lower the food is on the glycemic index. In addition, many instant oatmeal brands on the market today are not gluten-free—they contain oats that have been cross-contaminated with a tiny bit of wheat, rye, or barley. Be sure to choose certified gluten-free oatmeal for this dish.

Spinach and Gorgonzola Egg-White Omelet

This is a diet and comfort food. That may seem like an impossible combination, but in this case it is true. The quick and easy spinach filling comes from frozen spinach soufflé.

INGREDIENTS | SERVES 2

Nonstick butter-flavored cooking spray, as needed

1 (12-ounce) frozen spinach soufflé, defrosted

8 egg whites, well beaten

⅛ teaspoon ground nutmeg

1 teaspoon finely grated lemon zest

½ cup crumbled Gorgonzola cheese

The Versatile Omelet

The fantastic thing about an omelet is that you can stuff it with all kinds of ingredients. Various veggies, fruit, and cheeses and combinations thereof make exciting omelets. Try mixing some Cheddar cheese sauce and broccoli or some Brie and raspberries for your next omelet and enjoy the flavors!

1. Prepare a medium nonstick pan with cooking spray. Make sure the spinach soufflé is thoroughly defrosted.

2. Place pan over medium-high heat. Pour in beaten egg whites and sprinkle with nutmeg, lemon zest, and cheese. Let the egg set for 1–2 minutes. Spoon 1 cup spinach soufflé down the middle of the omelet. Reserve the rest for another use.

3. When the omelet starts to set, fold the outsides over the center. Cook until it reaches your desired level of firmness.

Tomato, Bell Pepper, and Feta Frittata

This frittata can be made for a quick and easy breakfast or a relaxed weekend brunch.

INGREDIENTS | SERVES 1

2 egg whites

1 large egg

2 tablespoons crumbled feta cheese

½ cup chopped tomato

¼ cup chopped green bell pepper

Nonstick butter-flavored cooking spray, as needed

Salt and ground black pepper, to taste

Healthy Egg Dish

Quiches taste great, but they are loaded with fat, cholesterol, and calories. Plus, the crust often has a high glycemic value. Frittatas are a GI-friendly and lighter option for a delicious and easy egg dish.

1. Place egg whites in a medium bowl. Add whole egg and whisk to combine.

2. Add feta, tomato, and bell pepper to eggs and whisk to combine.

3. Cook egg mixture over medium heat in a small skillet coated with cooking spray for 4 minutes or until eggs are firm. Do not stir.

4. Flip and cook the other side for 2 more minutes. Season with salt and pepper to taste.

Scrambled Eggs with Sausage and Jalapeño

This is a very pretty dish that is not only delicious for breakfast but is also good for lunch or a late supper. Be careful not to overly salt the dish—most sausage has quite a lot of salt in it, so taste first.

INGREDIENTS | SERVES 4

1 pound sweet Italian sausage

¼ cup water

1 tablespoon olive oil

2 red bell peppers, roasted and chopped

1 jalapeño pepper, seeded and minced

8 large eggs

¾ cup 2% milk

2 tablespoons chopped fresh flat-leaf parsley, for garnish

1. Cut sausage into ¼" coins. Place in a heavy frying pan with water and olive oil. Bring to a boil, then reduce to a simmer.

2. When sausage is brown, remove to a paper towel. Add bell peppers and jalapeño pepper and sauté over medium heat for 5 minutes.

3. While the peppers sauté, beat eggs and milk together vigorously in a large bowl. Add eggs to the pan and gently fold until puffed and moist.

4. Mix in reserved sausage, garnish with parsley, and serve hot.

Cottage Cheese Pancakes

This batter can be whipped up in a snap for tasty high-protein pancakes or waffles.

INGREDIENTS | SERVES 4

½ cup almond flour

¼ teaspoon salt

¼ cup olive oil

1 cup low-fat milk

½ teaspoon vanilla extract

6 large eggs

1 cup low-fat cottage cheese

Nonstick cooking spray, as needed

Blueberry Pancakes

Try adding a few handfuls of blueberries to your pancake batter. Blueberries are an excellent source of antioxidant phytonutrients, called anthocyanidins, which are responsible for the blue-red pigment seen in blueberries. Anthocyanidins help protect the body from harm from free radicals.

1. Blend all ingredients, except cooking spray, in a blender until smooth.

2. Spray a large pan with nonstick cooking spray and place over medium heat. Pour ¼-cup portions of batter onto hot pan to form pancakes. As the pan heats up, adjust the temperature to prevent the pancakes from becoming too dark.

3. Cook for 2–3 minutes per side until golden brown. Make the pancakes in small batches and, when done, cover to keep warm.

Sweet Potato Pancakes

You'll never look at pancakes the same way again once you taste this sweet potato variety! Sweet, smooth, and flavorful, this healthier option outdoes the refined favorite in every aspect.

INGREDIENTS | SERVES 10

Nonstick cooking spray, as needed
1 cup sweet potato purée
1 cup plain low-fat Greek-style yogurt
1 cup unsweetened applesauce
2 egg whites
2 whole large eggs
2 teaspoons vanilla extract
2 tablespoons Sucanat
¼ cup 100% gluten-free flour
1 teaspoon baking powder
1 teaspoon pumpkin pie spice
1 teaspoon ground cinnamon
2 tablespoons agave nectar

1. Coat a large nonstick skillet with cooking spray and place over medium heat.

2. In a large bowl, combine all ingredients, except agave nectar, and mix well.

3. Scoop batter onto preheated skillet, using approximately ½ cup batter per pancake. Cook for 2–3 minutes on each side, or until golden brown.

4. Remove from heat, plate, and drizzle pancakes with agave nectar.

Berry Almond Scones

These slightly sweet scones have a light texture with a soft crumb.
Try different types of fruit, such as strawberries or blackberries, in place of the blueberries.

INGREDIENTS | SERVES 8

3 cups blanched almond flour

¾ cup arrowroot starch or tapioca starch

½ teaspoon baking soda

¼ teaspoon salt

¼ cup coconut palm sugar or granulated sugar

⅓ cup butter or Spectrum Organic All Vegetable Shortening

1 large egg, slightly whisked

⅔ cup almond milk

1 teaspoon vanilla extract

½ teaspoon lemon juice or apple cider vinegar

1 cup fresh or frozen blueberries (do not defrost if frozen)

Traditional Scones versus Almond Flour Scones

Traditional scones are created by shaping the dough into a round loaf and slicing it before baking. These scones, however, are made in a cake pan and then sliced into triangles after they are cooked because almond flour dough is not quite thick enough to support itself baking without a pan. You could use a scone baking pan, but it's just as easy to bake the dough in a cake pan and then slice it.

1. Preheat oven to 350°F. Line a 9" cake pan with parchment paper and spritz with nonstick cooking spray.

2. In a large bowl, whisk together almond flour, arrowroot starch, baking soda, salt, and sugar. Use a fork and knife or a pastry cutter to cut butter or shortening evenly into flour mixture until it resembles small peas. Set aside.

3. In a small bowl mix together egg, almond milk, vanilla extract, and lemon juice or vinegar.

4. Add wet ingredients to dry ingredients and mix until thoroughly incorporated. Add blueberries and mix. Batter will be thick. Pour batter into the prepared cake pan and smooth the top with a spatula.

5. Bake for 25–30 minutes, until the edges are golden-brown and a toothpick inserted in the middle comes out mostly clean with few crumbs.

6. Remove from oven and set aside to cool for several minutes. Cut into 8 triangular scones.

Chestnut Flour Crepes

*Chestnut flour is sweet and nutty, making the most delicious crepes you could imagine.
You can stuff them with fruit and whipped cream, or with savory fillings.*

INGREDIENTS | SERVES 12

2 large eggs

1 cup milk

½ teaspoon salt

½ cup chestnut flour

½ cup rice flour

2 teaspoons granulated sugar (optional)

2 tablespoons butter, melted (plus more for pan)

Using Nonstick Sauté Pans

Nonstick pans take all the grief out of making crepes. However, even if your pan is quite new, it's important to use a bit of butter for insurance and extra flavor. Keep the pan well-buttered and you will have an almost foolproof method for making perfect crepes.

1. Blend eggs, milk, and salt in a food processor. With the motor on low, slowly add flours, stopping occasionally to scrape down the sides.

2. Add sugar if you are making sweet crepes with sweet filling; omit if you are going to fill them with savory delights.

3. Pour in melted butter, and process until well blended.

4. Add a dot of butter to a small nonstick sauté pan over medium heat. Pour batter by ½-cup portions into the pan. Tilt the pan to spread the batter thinly.

5. Cook crepes on medium heat, turning, until browned on both sides; place on waxed paper and sprinkle with a bit of rice flour to prevent them from sticking.

6. When the crepes are done, you can fill them right away or store them in the refrigerator or freezer for later use.

Corn Crepes

*As with the Chestnut Flour Crepes (see recipe in this chapter), you can make
these in advance and store them in the refrigerator or freezer.*

INGREDIENTS | SERVES 12

2 large eggs

1 cup milk or buttermilk

½ teaspoon salt, or to taste

1 cup corn flour

2 teaspoons granulated sugar (optional)

2 tablespoons butter, melted

Vegetable oil, as needed

Storing Crepes

To store crepes, simply put a bit of corn
flour on sheets of waxed paper and stack
the crepes individually. Then put the whole
thing in a plastic bag and store.

1. Place eggs, milk, and salt in a food processor and
   blend until smooth.

2. With the motor on low, slowly add flour and spoon in
   sugar if you are making sweet crepes. Scrape down the
   sides of the mixing bowl often. Add melted butter.

3. Heat a small nonstick pan over medium heat and add
   a teaspoonful of vegetable oil. Pour batter by ½-cup
   portions into the pan. Tilt the pan to spread the batter
   evenly. Fry on medium heat, turning once, until
   browned on both sides.

4. Place crepes on sheets of waxed paper that have been
   dusted with extra corn flour.

5. To store, place in a plastic bag in the refrigerator or
   freezer. You can stuff these with salsa, eggs, and
   chopped vegetables, or mashed fruit such as strawberries and bananas.

Banana Nut Pancakes

For this recipe, you can either slice the bananas onto the cakes or mash them and incorporate them into the batter.

INGREDIENTS | SERVES 4

½ cup milk

2 large eggs

1½ tablespoons butter, melted

1 medium banana, mashed

1 tablespoon baking powder

1 cup rice flour (or substitute corn, chickpea, or tapioca flour)

Nonstick cooking spray, as needed

1 cup coarsely chopped walnuts

1. In the bowl of a food processor, combine milk, eggs, butter, and banana. Slowly add baking powder and flour until incorporated. Do not overmix.

2. Prepare a medium pan or griddle with nonstick spray. Heat pan on medium. Pour in batter ½-cup at a time. Sprinkle nuts on top of each cake.

3. Turn when pancakes begin to bubble on top. Place on a warm platter. Serve with freshly whipped cream, extra sliced bananas, or the fruit of your choice.

Blueberry or Strawberry Pancakes

These classic pancakes are sure to please your family as well as your own taste buds.

INGREDIENTS | SERVES 4

½ pint blueberries or strawberries

1 tablespoon granulated sugar

1 teaspoon grated orange zest

½ cup milk

2 large eggs

1½ tablespoons butter, melted

1 tablespoon baking powder

1 cup rice flour (or substitute corn, chickpea, or tapioca flour)

Nonstick cooking spray, as needed

Freezing Fruit in Its Prime

There's nothing like blueberry pie in January, and not the fruit that comes loaded with sugar syrup in a can. When fresh blueberries are available, just rinse a quart and dry on paper towels. Place the berries on a cookie sheet in the freezer for 30 minutes and then put them in a plastic bag for future use.

1. In a large bowl, mix fruit, sugar, and orange zest. Mash with a potato masher or mortar and pestle.

2. In the bowl of a food processor, combine milk, eggs, and butter. Slowly add baking powder and flour until incorporated. Do not overmix.

3. Prepare a medium pan or griddle with nonstick spray. Heat pan on medium. Pour pancake batter by ½-cup portions into the pan and spoon some berries on top.

4. Turn when bubbles rise to the top of the cakes, and brown the other side. You will get some caramelization from the sugar and fruit—it's delicious. Top with more berries and whipped cream to serve, if desired.

Egg-and-Cheese-Stuffed Tomatoes

This is a fine way to use up the end-of-summer tomatoes in your garden.

INGREDIENTS | SERVES 4

8 medium tomatoes

¼ cup butter

2 cloves garlic, minced

1 teaspoon salt

1 teaspoon ground black pepper

1½ teaspoons ground paprika

1 teaspoon dried oregano

1 teaspoon ground cumin

8 large eggs

½ cup grated Monterey jack or Cheddar cheese

8 teaspoons gluten-free corn bread crumbs

Priceless Heirlooms

There are good tomatoes in the supermarket and good tomatoes in cans, but the best tomatoes are homegrown. Recently there has been a trend toward growing ancient varieties of tomato. These "heirlooms," as they are called, have more flavor—having sweetness paired with acid—than ordinary tomatoes do. You can buy the seeds and grow them yourself, and some green markets have them too.

1. Cut off the tops of the tomatoes, core, and use a melon baller to scoop out seeds and pulp. Place tomatoes on a baking sheet covered with parchment paper or sprayed with nonstick spray.

2. Preheat oven to 350°F.

3. In a small pan, heat butter on medium and sauté garlic until fragrant. While it's cooking, mix together salt, black pepper, paprika, oregano, and cumin in a small bowl.

4. Rub the insides of the tomatoes with ½ the spice mixture. Spoon the butter and garlic mixture inside the tomatoes. Sprinkle with remaining spice mixture, reserving a bit for seasoning the eggs.

5. Break an egg into each tomato. Sprinkle with reserved spice mixture. Loosely spoon cheese over the eggs, then sprinkle 1 teaspoon corn bread crumbs over each tomato.

6. Bake for 20 minutes. The tomatoes should still be firm, the eggs soft, the cheese melted, and the bread crumbs browned.

Shirred Eggs with Crumbled Cheddar Topping

These eggs are so appealing—and super-simple to make. For an extra touch of flavor, you can place a thin slice of tomato in the bottom of each ramekin.

INGREDIENTS | SERVES 6

Nonstick cooking spray, as needed
12 extra-large eggs
Salt and ground black pepper, to taste
¼ cup butter
¾ cup grated Cheddar cheese

An Elegant Touch

If you are having a crowd of people to brunch, place ramekins on a baking sheet and bake for 10 minutes. Then, serve with a big bowl of fruit on the side. You can use glass custard cups, but individual ramekins made of white porcelain are more elegant.

1. Preheat oven to 350°F. Prepare 12 small (4-ounce) ramekins or 6 larger (6-ounce) ones with nonstick spray. Place the ramekins on a baking sheet. Break 1 egg into each of 12 or 2 eggs into each of 6 large ramekins.

2. Sprinkle the eggs with salt and pepper and dot with butter. Sprinkle with Cheddar cheese.

3. Bake for 8–12 minutes, or to desired doneness. Serve immediately.

Mini Quiches

*Mini Quiches are perfect as breakfast on the go or as a wonderful cocktail party snack.
To vary the ingredients, try using Cheddar cheese instead of Jarlsberg,
and chopped cooked bacon instead of prosciutto or ham.*

INGREDIENTS | SERVES 12

Nonstick cooking spray, as needed

1 (16-ounce) package gluten-free pie crust mix

2 large eggs

½ cup grated Jarlsberg cheese

¼ cup minced prosciutto or smoked ham

⅔ cup heavy cream

⅛ teaspoon grated nutmeg

2 tablespoons minced fresh chives

Freshly ground black pepper, to taste

1. Preheat oven to 325°F. Spray a 12-cup mini-muffin pan with nonstick spray.

2. Prepare the pie crust mix according to box directions. Roll out thinly. With the floured rim of a juice glass or a 2" biscuit cutter, cut dough into 12 rounds and line the muffin cups with dough.

3. Pulse the remaining ingredients in a food processor until combined.

4. Fill the cups ¾ full with the cheese mixture.

5. Bake for about 10 minutes, or until set. Let rest for 5 minutes. Carefully lift the quiches from the cups. Serve warm.

CHAPTER 8

Lunch

Asian Sesame Lettuce Wraps

Lettuce wraps make a light and tasty lunch as well as a fun finger food for appetizers.

INGREDIENTS | SERVES 4

1 tablespoon vegetable oil

2 cloves garlic, minced

2 green onions, chopped

2 tablespoons grated gingerroot

1 pound ground chicken

½ cup gluten-free soy sauce

1 (5-ounce) can water chestnuts, chopped

1 teaspoon crushed red pepper flakes

½ cup chopped fresh cilantro

1 tablespoon sesame seeds

1 large head Boston or butter lettuce, leaves separated

1. Heat oil in a large pan; add garlic, green onion, and ginger and sauté about 3 minutes.

2. Add ground chicken to the pan and additional oil if needed. Then add soy sauce, water chestnuts, and red pepper flakes. Cook until chicken is brown and crumbling apart, about 5 minutes.

3. When chicken is cooked, add chopped cilantro and sesame seeds immediately. Serve chicken mixture in a serving bowl with lettuce leaves on the side for scooping.

Vegan Option

For a vegetarian-friendly lettuce wrap, use tofu instead of ground chicken. The tofu will take on the flavor of the soy sauce and ginger. Firm or extra-firm tofu will hold up better in this recipe than soft tofu.

Chicken Breast with Scallions, Snap Peas, and Beans

The snap peas and white beans add to the protein in this recipe and provide a shot of energy that will last for hours. Aside from being a convenient one-pot meal, this is a delectable dish.

INGREDIENTS | SERVES 2

½ pound boneless, skinless chicken breasts

Salt and ground black pepper, to taste

2 tablespoons olive oil

2 cloves garlic, chopped

10 scallions, chopped

1 cup chopped snap peas

1 tablespoon chopped fresh rosemary or 1 teaspoon dried rosemary

4 fresh basil leaves, or 1 teaspoon dried basil

2 tablespoons dry white vermouth

1 cup canned whole tomatoes, drained

1 (15-ounce) can white beans, drained and rinsed

1 teaspoon crushed red pepper flakes, or to taste

1. Cut chicken into large chunks; sprinkle with salt and pepper. In a Dutch oven, heat olive oil over medium heat. Add garlic and chicken, and sauté for 3–4 minutes.

2. Add scallions and snap peas; toss, and cook for 4 minutes.

3. Stir in remaining ingredients; cover and simmer for 10 minutes, and serve.

Spiced Stuffed Peppers

Green peppers are divine, but red, yellow, and orange peppers have more vitamin C. You can mix leftover veggies in with the rice or lentils for an impromptu supper.

INGREDIENTS | SERVES 2

2 tablespoons olive oil

¼ cup finely chopped red onion

1 clove garlic, minced

2 sprigs fresh parsley, minced

1 teaspoon coriander seed, cracked

Tabasco sauce, to taste

1 teaspoon dried thyme

Salt and ground black pepper, to taste

1 cup cooked basmati rice

2 extra-large bell peppers

Nonstick cooking spray, as needed

2 cups canned puréed tomatoes

2 tablespoons grated Parmesan cheese

1. Heat olive oil on medium-low in a medium pan. Stir in onions and garlic, and sauté for 4 minutes. Add parsley, coriander, Tabasco, thyme, salt, and pepper. When well mixed, spoon in rice, stirring to coat with oil, herbs, and spices.

2. Preheat oven to 350°F. Lightly spray a shallow baking pan with cooking spray.

3. Cut each pepper in half lengthwise, and remove stems and seeds. Fill with rice mixture. Pour puréed tomatoes over the top. Sprinkle with Parmesan cheese.

4. Bake for 35 minutes.

Veggie Burger Sliders

These mini burgers are delicious as a quick weeknight meal, but they also make great party appetizers if you want to double or triple the recipe to feed a crowd.

INGREDIENTS | SERVES 4

1 (15-ounce) can red kidney beans, drained and rinsed

½ cup dried bread crumbs (or more if beans are very wet)

½ cup chopped red onion

2 tablespoons Worcestershire sauce

2 tablespoons barbecue sauce

1 large egg

1 teaspoon dried oregano, rosemary, thyme, basil, or sage

Salt and ground black pepper, to taste

½ cup brown rice, cooked

2 tablespoons canola oil

1. Pulse all ingredients except rice and canola oil in a food processor or blender. Transfer to a large bowl.

2. Add brown rice to bean mixture and stir to mix well.

3. Form into mini burger patties.

4. Heat oil to 300°F in a large skillet. Fry burgers on each side until very hot. Serve on gluten-free rolls, wrapped in lettuce, or plain.

The Praises of Brown Rice

Unlike white rice, which is rice with its outer layers removed, brown rice has lost only the hard outer hull of the grain when it gets to the store. As a result, brown rice contains many more nutrients than its more processed relative. Also, the fiber in brown rice decreases your risk for colon cancer and helps lower cholesterol!

Grilled Pork and Mango Salsa Sandwich

One of the nicest cuts of pork is the tenderloin. It cooks quickly and pairs well with fruit such as mangoes, pineapples, apples, and peaches.

INGREDIENTS | SERVES 4

1 (12-ounce) package gluten-free corn bread mix

1 (1-pound) pork tenderloin, trimmed

2 tablespoons gluten-free soy sauce

Salt and ground black pepper, to taste

2 tablespoons peanut oil

½ cup Mango Salsa (see recipe in Chapter 13)

1. Prepare the corn bread according to package directions. Bake, and cut into 8 squares (2" × 2").

2. Sprinkle pork tenderloin with soy sauce, salt, and pepper.

3. Heat a large, heavy frying pan over medium heat and add peanut oil. Sauté pork for 8 minutes per side or until medium, turning frequently. When done, let rest for 8–10 minutes. Slice thinly on a diagonal.

4. Place 2 pieces of corn bread on each serving plate. Stack slices of pork on each. Top with Mango Salsa.

Thanksgiving Wraps

You don't have to wait for Turkey Day leftovers to enjoy these!

INGREDIENTS | SERVES 6

2 cups diced cooked turkey

1 medium stalk celery, minced

½ cup red seedless grapes, halved

2 tablespoons minced red onion

¼ cup dried cranberries

6 tablespoons low-fat mayonnaise

1 teaspoon dried thyme

Salt and ground black pepper, to taste

12 large romaine lettuce leaves

1. Toss together all ingredients except lettuce in a large bowl.

2. Lay out lettuce leaves, add turkey filling, and roll them up.

Cranberry Additions

Dried cranberries make a tasty addition to many everyday foods. Add them to cereal, trail mix, oatmeal cookies, chocolate chip cookies, and salads for a sweet and tart surprise.

Grilled Vegetable and Cheese Panini

Panini are grilled sandwiches usually stuffed with vegetables, cheese, and grilled meat. They are grilled in a panini press or in a frying pan with a heavy weight on top to squish them down. You can use a heavy frying pan or foil-covered brick as the weight.

INGREDIENTS | SERVES 2

2 baby eggplants, thinly sliced

½ yellow summer squash, cut into ¼" coins

¼ cup Italian Dressing (see recipe in Chapter 12)

1 medium red bell pepper, cored and seeded

2 teaspoons grated Parmesan cheese

4 slices gluten-free Italian bread

2 thin slices Muenster cheese

2 teaspoons crumbled Gorgonzola cheese

Oil, as needed

1. Preheat grill on medium. Brush eggplant and squash with about half of the dressing.

2. Grill eggplant and squash on each side. Grill bell pepper, turning until charred on all sides. Place pepper, while still hot, in a plastic bag. Let cool, then peel off skin. Slice into strips. Sprinkle veggies with Parmesan cheese and set aside.

3. Spread both sides of each bread slice with remaining Italian Dressing. Load 2 slices with vegetables and Muenster and Gorgonzola cheese, and top with remaining bread slices.

4. Lightly oil a large frying pan or panini press and heat on medium. If using a frying pan, place a second pan or foil-covered brick on top of sandwiches in the frying pan. Toast the sandwiches on medium heat until well browned. Turn if using a frying pan.

5. Cut sandwiches and serve piping hot.

Bacon, Kale, and Sun-Dried Tomato Quiche

This lovely crustless quiche makes a beautiful dish that's fancy enough for company. Spinach, Swiss chard, or other dark leafy greens can be substituted for the kale.

INGREDIENTS | SERVES 4

Nonstick cooking spray, as needed

5 large eggs

1 (14-ounce) can unsweetened coconut milk

½ teaspoon salt

½ teaspoon ground black pepper

6 ounces bacon or turkey bacon

1–2 tablespoons olive oil

1 medium sweet onion, diced

3 cups chopped fresh kale

½ cup chopped sun-dried tomatoes

Use What You Have on Hand

Don't have bacon? Use ½ pound of bulk sausage or ground beef. Don't have kale? Use a bag of fresh baby spinach instead. Don't have sun-dried tomatoes? Use a chopped red bell pepper instead. Don't need to worry about dairy? Add ½ cup shredded Cheddar or mozzarella to the whisked eggs.

1. Preheat oven to 350°F. Grease a 9" deep-dish pie pan with nonstick cooking spray.

2. In a large bowl whisk together eggs, coconut milk, salt, and pepper. Set aside.

3. In a large heavy-bottomed skillet cook bacon on medium-high heat to desired crispiness. Remove from pan and drain on a plate lined with paper towels.

4. Remove and discard most of the bacon fat from the pan, reserving about 1 tablespoon. Add olive oil to the pan and heat for 1–2 minutes, until sizzling. Add onion and cook over medium-high heat for 3–5 minutes, until translucent. Add kale and cook for 3–4 minutes, until bright green and slightly wilted.

5. Crumble bacon and sprinkle over the bottom of the prepared pie pan. Add cooked onion, chopped sun-dried tomatoes, and kale to pie pan and spread out evenly. Pour egg mixture over cooked ingredients. Place the pie pan on a large baking sheet to catch spills while baking.

6. Bake for 35–45 minutes, until the center of the quiche is set and a knife inserted in the middle comes out clean. Allow quiche to cool for 10–15 minutes before serving.

Frittata with Asparagus, Cheddar, and Monterey Jack

Some matches are made in heaven, and asparagus with eggs and cheese is a divine combination.

INGREDIENTS | SERVES 4

1 (10-ounce) box frozen chopped asparagus

Nonstick cooking spray, as needed

2 tablespoons butter

6 large eggs

1 cup grated Cheddar cheese

¼ cup shredded Monterey jack or pepper jack cheese

1 teaspoon grated lemon zest

Salt and ground black pepper, to taste

Use Up Your Leftovers

The frittata is a staple in Italy—putting a lot of eggs together with leftover or fresh vegetables is a fine way of using every precious bit of food. A frittata can be jazzed up with a variety of herbs and cheeses. The only thing to remember about frittatas is that just about anything goes!

1. Cook the asparagus according to package directions and drain. If using fresh asparagus, trim off woody ends and boil for 10 minutes; drain and chop.

2. Prepare an ovenproof 12" pan with nonstick spray, then add butter and melt over medium-high heat.

3. In a medium bowl, beat eggs. Mix in cheeses, lemon zest, and salt and pepper.

4. Pour egg mixture into pan, distribute asparagus, and reduce heat to low; cook slowly for 10–15 minutes. Preheat broiler.

5. Place pan under broiler for 10 seconds, or until nicely browned.

Shrimp and Lobster Salad

Try using different citrus fruit and mixing in different vegetables.
And if you like cilantro, use that instead of parsley.

INGREDIENTS | SERVES 4

1 cup mayonnaise

1 teaspoon gluten-free Dijon mustard

Juice of ½ lime

1 teaspoon grated lime zest

1 teaspoon gluten-free soy sauce

1 tablespoon chili sauce

1 teaspoon minced garlic

Salt and ground black pepper, to taste

Meat of 1 small (1½-pound) lobster, cooked and roughly chopped

½ pound medium shrimp, peeled, deveined, and cooked

2 tablespoons snipped fresh dill weed

2 tablespoons chopped fresh flat-leaf parsley

1 tablespoon capers

4 cups shredded lettuce

1. In a medium bowl, mix together mayonnaise, mustard, lime juice, lime zest, soy sauce, chili sauce, minced garlic, and salt and pepper.

2. Just before serving, mix together prepared sauce and seafood. Garnish with dill weed and parsley, sprinkle with capers, and serve over a bed of lettuce.

Capers

These tiny berries are pickled in brine or packed in salt. The islands of the Mediterranean are lush with the bushes that produce them and they are used in profusion in many fish, meat, and salad dishes. The French love them, as do the Italians, Greeks, Sardinians, and Maltese. Try some in a butter sauce over a piece of fresh striped bass and you'll understand their popularity.

Stuffed Portobello Mushrooms with Roasted Tomatoes and Quinoa

You can substitute rice for quinoa if you prefer; however, you get a nice nutty flavor from the quinoa.

INGREDIENTS | SERVES 4

4 portobello mushrooms, about 4–5" in diameter, stemmed and brushed off

16 cherry tomatoes, cut in half

¼ cup olive oil

1 tablespoon minced garlic

2 cups cooked quinoa

¼ cup finely chopped walnuts (almonds or pecans are fine)

¼ cup butter or margarine, melted

1 teaspoon ground turmeric

Salt, to taste

Crushed red pepper flakes, to taste

¼ cup capers (optional)

¼ cup golden raisins (optional)

1 teaspoon grated lemon zest (optional)

1. Preheat oven to 350°F. Place the mushrooms on a well-greased baking sheet. Set aside.

2. Place tomatoes on another baking sheet and toss with olive oil and garlic. Roast in oven for 20 minutes or until soft.

3. Mix together roasted tomatoes, cooked quinoa, nuts, butter or margarine, and seasonings. Add optional ingredients if desired. Spoon into mushrooms.

4. Bake for 30 minutes or until hot and soft.

Do You Know Quinoa?

Rich, nutrient-filled quinoa is considered a supergrain, though it is not really a grain but the starchy seed of a plant related to spinach. The protein in quinoa is more complete than that of other grains, and contains the amino acid lysine, as does buckwheat and amaranth. The quality of quinoa's protein is equivalent to that of milk.

Indian Vegetable Cakes

This is a great way to get kids to eat their veggies. A nonstick pan helps prevent sticking. Sour cream makes a good garnish.

INGREDIENTS | SERVES 4–6

1 tablespoon olive oil

1 (10-ounce) package frozen chopped spinach, thawed and squeezed of excess moisture

½ (10-ounce) box frozen baby peas, thawed

½ bunch scallions, chopped

1 teaspoon gluten-free curry powder

Salt, to taste

Hot pepper sauce, to taste

¼ cup gluten-free cornmeal

5 extra-large eggs, well beaten

½ cup grated Parmesan cheese

1. Heat olive oil in a large nonstick pan over medium heat.

2. In a large bowl mix together all ingredients except Parmesan cheese and form into patties.

3. Drop patties, 3 to 4 at a time, into the pan and fry until delicately browned. Turn and sprinkle with cheese. Let cook for 2–3 minutes for cheese to melt and second side to brown.

Thai Chicken with Peanut Dipping Sauce

For satay recipes, chicken (or other meats) should be grilled over hot coals. You can use tender beef instead of chicken in this recipe—the marinade is good with any meat.

INGREDIENTS | SERVES 4

For the chicken:

1½ pounds boneless, skinless chicken breast

½ cup gluten-free soy sauce

2 teaspoons Thai red chili paste, or to taste

2 tablespoons minced gingerroot

1 tablespoon sesame oil

2 tablespoons dry sherry

For the sauce:

½ cup unsweetened coconut milk

1 cup dry-roasted peanuts

1 tablespoon lemon or lime juice

1 tablespoon dark brown sugar, or more to taste

1 tablespoon gluten-free dark soy sauce

½ teaspoon chili oil, or to taste

2 tablespoons peanut oil

2 tablespoons finely chopped sweet onion

2 cloves garlic, minced

1. Set 12 (10") skewers to soak in water to cover for at least 40 minutes (if using wooden skewers). Rinse chicken, pat dry, and cut it into bite-sized pieces.

2. In a large bowl, mix together chicken marinade ingredients and add the chicken. Cover and marinate for 2 hours.

3. While the chicken is marinating, prepare the dipping sauce. In a food processor or blender, combine coconut milk, peanuts, lemon or lime juice, brown sugar, soy sauce, and chili oil. Process until very smooth.

4. Heat peanut oil in a large saucepan. Add onion and garlic and cook over medium heat until just soft, about 3 minutes.

5. Pour peanut mixture into pan and mix well. Heat on low, but do not boil. Preheat grill to medium-high.

6. String chicken onto skewers and grill for 4–5 minutes per side. Serve with the warmed dipping sauce.

CHAPTER 9

Dinner

Poached Chicken with Pears and Herbs

Any seasonal fresh fruit will make a dish special. If you have some fruit brandy, a splash will also add to the flavor. Double this recipe for company.

INGREDIENTS | SERVES 2

1 large ripe pear, peeled, cored, and cut into chunks

2 shallots, minced

½ cup dry white wine

1 teaspoon dried rosemary or 1 tablespoon chopped fresh rosemary

1 teaspoon dried thyme or 1 tablespoon chopped fresh thyme

Salt and ground black pepper, to taste

2½ pounds boneless, skinless chicken breasts

1. Prepare the poaching liquid: In a large saucepan, combine pear, shallots, wine, rosemary, and thyme. Bring to a boil.

2. Salt and pepper chicken and add to saucepan. Reduce heat to a simmer and cook slowly for 10 minutes.

3. Spoon pear on top of chicken and serve.

Golden Sautéed Diver Scallops

This recipe calls for caramelizing the scallops—an amazing way to add flavor and texture to the sweet scallops.

INGREDIENTS | SERVES 4

½ cup corn flour

2 tablespoons granulated sugar

1 teaspoon salt

½ teaspoon ground white pepper

1½ pounds large diver scallops, each about 2" wide

2 tablespoons unsalted butter

2 tablespoons olive oil

1. On a sheet of waxed paper or a shallow dish, mix flour, sugar, salt, and pepper. Roll scallops in flour mixture.

2. Heat butter and oil in a large skillet over medium-high heat. Add scallops and cook for 2–3 minutes per side, until opaque. Watch carefully, as they will brown quickly. Serve with any of your favorite sauces.

Lemon Chicken

This citrusy chicken with fresh herbs is flavorful without being too sour—it's the perfect amount of lemon.

INGREDIENTS | SERVES 4–6

⅓ cup lemon juice

2 tablespoons grated lemon zest

3 cloves garlic, minced

2 tablespoons chopped fresh thyme

2 tablespoons chopped fresh rosemary

2 tablespoons olive oil

1 teaspoon salt

1 teaspoon ground black pepper

3 pounds bone-in chicken thighs

1. To make the marinade, combine lemon juice, lemon zest, garlic, thyme, rosemary, olive oil, salt, and pepper in a small bowl.

2. Place chicken in a large bowl and pour marinade on top. Let marinate in the refrigerator for 2 hours.

3. Preheat oven to 425°F. Place marinated chicken in a single layer in a large baking dish. Spoon leftover marinade over top of chicken.

4. Bake until chicken is completely cooked through, about 50 minutes. The internal temperature should read 175°F.

Moroccan Chicken Tagine

This tantalizing one-pot meal is bursting with spices, fresh herbs, and Moroccan flavor.

INGREDIENTS | SERVES 6

¼ cup cooking oil

1 large onion, thinly sliced

2 cloves garlic, minced

2 teaspoons chopped fresh cilantro

¼ teaspoon ground cinnamon

1 teaspoon ground ginger

1 teaspoon ground cumin

½ teaspoon ground black pepper

Pinch ground cayenne pepper

Salt, to taste

1 large tomato, chopped

3 cups canned chickpeas, drained and rinsed

½ cup water

1 (5-pound) whole chicken, cut into serving pieces

1 cup black olives, pitted

1. Add oil to a large pan over medium-high heat. Add onion to hot oil and cook, stirring occasionally, for about 5 minutes or until tender. Add garlic, cilantro, and spices. Cook for 1 minute, stirring continuously. Add tomato, chickpeas, and water, and bring to a boil.

2. Season chicken pieces with salt. Place chicken in sauce. Reduce heat to medium-low, cover, and simmer for 35 minutes. Add olives and continue cooking for 10 more minutes.

Sirloin Steak with Tomato Salad

This simple, flavorful supper makes a wonderful summertime meal.

INGREDIENTS | SERVES 2

½ pound lean, boneless sirloin steak, thinly sliced

2 tablespoons plus 2 teaspoons French Dressing (see recipe in Chapter 12)

Salt and ground black pepper, to taste

1 teaspoon olive oil

1 large ripe tomato, quartered

1. Marinate steak in 2 tablespoons dressing for 20 minutes. Sprinkle with salt and pepper.

2. Heat a large frying pan to medium-high heat and add oil. Quickly sear steak slices on both sides for about 3–4 minutes.

3. Pile steak on 2 plates. Top each with tomato, drizzle with remaining dressing, and season with salt and pepper to taste. Serve.

Beef Tenderloin with Chimichurri

This is simple to make for an easy weeknight meal or perfect for a sophisticated gourmet dinner party.

INGREDIENTS | SERVES 2

1 cup parsley
3 cloves garlic
¼ cup capers, drained
2 tablespoons red wine vinegar
1 teaspoon gluten-free Dijon mustard
2 tablespoons olive oil
Salt and ground black pepper, to taste
2 (5-ounce) beef tenderloins

1. Preheat grill to medium-high, or heat a grill pan over medium-high heat.

2. In a blender or food processor, combine parsley, garlic, capers, vinegar, mustard, and oil. Season with salt and pepper as desired.

3. Grill tenderloins to medium-rare, about 3–4 minutes per side, until the internal temperature reaches 140°F. Serve with chimichurri sauce.

Rosemary Pork Chops with Apples and Raisins

Apple and rosemary pair perfectly with pork chops.

INGREDIENTS | SERVES 4

4 boneless pork loin chops

2 teaspoons olive oil, divided

2 tablespoons chopped fresh rosemary

¼ teaspoon salt

¼ teaspoon ground black pepper

1 medium Granny Smith apple, cored and quartered

¼ cup golden raisins

¾ cup red wine

Nonstick cooking spray, as needed

1. Rub pork chops lightly with 1 teaspoon olive oil. Combine rosemary, salt, and pepper, and rub evenly on both sides of pork chops.

2. Heat a medium skillet on medium and add remaining oil. Cook apple and raisins for 4 minutes, stirring constantly.

3. Add half the wine and cook until the liquid evaporates, stirring constantly. Add remaining wine and cook on medium-low heat for 15 minutes.

4. In a large skillet treated with cooking spray, cook pork chops over medium heat for 6–8 minutes on each side (depending on the thickness of the chops). Serve chops with apple mixture.

Winter Root Vegetable Soufflé

This recipe puts to good use all the wonderful root vegetables available in the winter months and provides an alternative to simply mashing them with butter. If you're looking for a lighter option, you can substitute nonfat milk for the 2% in this recipe.

INGREDIENTS | SERVES 4

Nonstick cooking spray, as needed

½ large Vidalia onion, cut into large chunks

2 medium carrots, peeled and chopped

2 medium parsnips, peeled and chopped

2 baby turnips, peeled and cut into pieces

1 teaspoon salt

4 eggs, separated, whites reserved

1 teaspoon dried sage

2 tablespoons chopped fresh flat-leaf parsley

1 tablespoon gluten-free flour

½ teaspoon Tabasco sauce, or to taste

½ cup 2% milk

Soufflé Tip

It's okay to have a soufflé flop, especially in the case of cheese and vegetable soufflés. A dessert soufflé should never fall. If, as directed, you start the soufflé with the oven at 400°F and then reduce the temperature, you are more likely to produce a high soufflé!

1. Preheat oven to 400°F. Prepare a 2-quart soufflé dish with nonstick spray.

2. Place vegetables in a large pot of cold water, add salt, and cover. Bring to a boil; reduce heat and simmer until veggies are very tender.

3. Drain vegetables and let cool slightly. Place in a blender and purée. With the blender running on medium speed, add egg yolks, 1 at a time. Then add sage, parsley, flour, Tabasco sauce, and milk. Pour into a large bowl.

4. Beat egg whites until stiff. Fold egg whites into the purée. Pour into the prepared soufflé dish.

5. Bake for 20 minutes at 400°F. Reduce heat to 350°F and bake for 20 minutes more. Don't worry if your soufflé flops just before serving; it will still be light and delicious.

Asian Sesame-Crusted Scallops

Scallops can be grilled, broiled, or sautéed. Try to get really big scallops—called sea scallops. They are very sweet and velvety in texture. These are delicious as an appetizer for 4 or as a main course for 2.

INGREDIENTS | SERVES 2

2 cups shredded napa cabbage

1 large ripe tomato, sliced

¼ cup gluten-free soy sauce

2 tablespoons sesame oil

Juice of ½ lime

1" piece gingerroot, peeled and minced

½ pound diver scallops (3–4 per person)

1 large egg, beaten

½ cup sesame seeds

2 tablespoons peanut oil

Salt and ground black pepper, to taste

1. Arrange cabbage and tomato slices on 2 serving plates. In a small bowl, mix together soy sauce, sesame oil, lime juice, and minced ginger to create sauce.

2. Rinse scallops and pat dry on paper towels. Dip scallops in beaten egg. Spread sesame seeds on waxed paper or a shallow plate, and roll scallops in them to cover.

3. Heat peanut oil in a large nonstick frying pan over medium heat. Sear scallops until browned on both sides and heated through. Do not overcook, or they will get tough. Arrange scallops over cabbage and tomatoes; season with salt and pepper. Drizzle with the sauce.

Almond Flour Chicken Pot Pie

*This savory pie is topped with almond flour pastry dough. If you prefer,
you can make a batch of gluten-free biscuits and top the pie with that instead.*

INGREDIENTS | SERVES 6–8

Nonstick cooking spray, as needed

Filling:

2 tablespoons olive oil

⅓ cup blanched almond flour or 3 tablespoons arrowroot starch

½ teaspoon salt

1 teaspoon ground black pepper

2 cups Chicken Broth (see recipe in Chapter 11) or the cooking liquid from chicken

2½ cups chopped cooked chicken (or the cooked meat from a small roasted chicken)

1 (15-ounce) can peas and carrots, drained

Pastry:

1½ cups blanched almond flour

¼ teaspoon sea salt

2 tablespoons olive oil

1 large egg, beaten

1. Preheat oven to 350°F. Grease a 9" deep-dish pie pan with nonstick cooking spray.

2. In a large saucepan, heat olive oil on medium. Add almond flour or arrowroot starch to the oil. Stir and cook for several minutes. Add salt, pepper, and broth. Stir until the broth has thickened into a sauce that will coat the back of a spoon. Stir in chicken and vegetables. Pour filling into prepared pie pan.

3. Make the pastry: In a medium bowl stir together almond flour and salt. Mix in olive oil and egg to form a thick dough. Place the dough between two sheets of parchment paper or plastic wrap that have been dusted with arrowroot starch. Roll into a 9" circle (about ¼" thick). Gently place pastry over chicken filling. It doesn't have to be perfect and you can patch the dough as necessary. If you have extra dough, you can roll it out and cut with cookie cutters into small stars or leaves.

4. Place pan on a baking sheet to prevent spills while baking. Bake for 30–40 minutes until the crust is golden brown and the sauce is bubbling up around the sides. Let the pot pie rest for at least 10 minutes before serving.

Orange Sesame Vinaigrette

A heavy meal like chicken pot pie needs a light side dish or first course, and a simple green salad is a great choice. To top the salad, make homemade Orange Sesame Vinaigrette by adding the following to a glass jar: ½ cup orange juice, 3 tablespoons olive oil, 1 tablespoon sesame oil, 1 tablespoon honey, and freshly ground salt and pepper. Cover jar and shake vigorously to combine. Drizzle a few tablespoons of vinaigrette over each salad.

Hearty Pot Roast

This is a traditional holiday dish, but is also great on ordinary weekends too.
Serve with mashed potatoes and winter vegetables.

INGREDIENTS | SERVES 6

1 (4-pound) top or bottom round beef roast

4 cloves garlic, slivered

1 teaspoon salt

1 teaspoon ground black pepper

Pinch ground cinnamon

Pinch ground nutmeg

1 slice bacon, cut into pieces

4 shallots, peeled and halved

2 red onions, peeled and quartered

¼ cup cognac

2 cups dry red wine

1 cup Beef Broth (see recipe in Chapter 11)

1 teaspoon dried thyme

4 whole cloves

¼ cup cornstarch mixed with ⅓ cup cold water until smooth

1. Make several cuts in the meat and put slivers of garlic in each. Rub the roast with salt, pepper, cinnamon, and nutmeg.

2. Heat bacon on medium in the bottom of a Dutch oven. Remove the bacon before it gets crisp, and brown the roast. Surround the roast with shallots and onions. Add cognac, wine, broth, thyme, and cloves.

3. Cover the pan and place in a 250°F oven for 5–6 hours. When the meat is done, place the roast on a warm platter. Add the cornstarch-water mixture to the pan juices and bring to a boil, stirring until thickened. Slice the roast. Serve the sauce over the pot roast with the vegetables surrounding the meat.

A Robust, Delectable Pot Roast

Slow cookers are excellent for cooking a pot roast. Either a top or bottom round is great. Chuck tends to be stringy. Trim the roast well, but do leave a bit of fat on it. You can also marinate a pot roast overnight in red wine and herbs. That will give you a deliciously tender piece of meat.

Curried Shrimp with Avocados

Adapting Asian flavors to American dishes can produce delightful meals such as this.
Quick and simply made, it's great as a light supper served with rice.

INGREDIENTS | SERVES 4

¾ cup mayonnaise

2 teaspoons gluten-free curry powder

Juice of 1 large lime

1 teaspoon hot chili oil or hot pepper
sauce such as Tabasco

½ pound raw medium shrimp, peeled
and deveined

4 medium ripe avocados, halved, peeled,
and pitted

Nonstick cooking spray, as needed

Hungarian sweet or hot paprika, to taste

Dry-roasted peanuts, for garnish

1. Preheat oven to 350°F.

2. In a medium bowl, mix together mayonnaise, curry powder, lime juice, and hot chili oil. Chop shrimp and mix with mayonnaise sauce.

3. Place avocado halves in a baking dish coated with nonstick spray. Spoon shrimp and sauce mixture into avocados. Sprinkle with paprika and peanuts.

4. Bake the shrimp-stuffed avocados for 20 minutes. You can vary this by adding chopped tart apple, pineapple, or red grapes.

How Hot Is Too Hot?

Any supermarket has dozens of bottles of various kinds of hot sauce, from Jamaican to Chinese to African to, of course, Asian. The degrees of heat and other flavorings such as garlic, ginger, etc., vary. However, for the flavors of the food to come through, use only as much as you find adds piquancy—don't burn your tongue or you will kill valuable taste buds.

Herb-Stuffed Veal Chops

This recipe calls for thick-cut chops. You can use double rib chops with a pocket for the aromatic herbs and vegetables. These can be grilled or sautéed.

INGREDIENTS | SERVES 4

½ cup minced shallots

2 tablespoons chopped fresh rosemary

2 teaspoons dried basil or 1 tablespoon chopped fresh basil

½ teaspoon ground coriander

2 tablespoons unsalted butter

1 teaspoon salt, plus extra for seasoning chops

Ground black pepper, to taste

4 veal rib chops, 1½–2" thick, with a pocket cut from the outside edge toward the bone in each

¼ cup olive oil

1. In a medium sauté pan over medium heat, sauté shallots and herbs in butter until tender, about 5–7 minutes. Add 1 teaspoon salt and pepper.

2. Stuff chops with herb mixture. Rub chops with olive oil, salt, and pepper.

3. Using an outdoor grill or oven broiler, sear the chops over high heat. Reduce heat to medium and cook for 4–5 minutes per side for medium chops or rare chops, depending on the thickness.

Grilled Portobello Mushrooms

These big, meaty mushrooms are great sliced over salad, stuffed, or chopped and stirred into sauce.

INGREDIENTS | SERVES 4

4 large (4–5" in diameter) portobello mushrooms, stems removed and caps brushed off
1 cup balsamic vinaigrette
Salt and ground black pepper, to taste

Mushrooms and Protein

Mushrooms are not really high in protein but they are filling. The large portobello mushrooms are great for grilling or stuffing with all kinds of goodies. They make excellent bases for rice, quinoa, eggs, and vegetables.

1. Marinate mushrooms in vinaigrette for 1–2 hours, covered, in the refrigerator.

2. Preheat grill to glowing coals, or set your gas grill to low.

3. Season mushrooms with salt and pepper. Grill mushrooms about 5–6 minutes per side, then slice and serve.

Stuffed Eggplant with Ricotta and Spices

This dish is also known as Eggplant Sicilian. It freezes beautifully and is delicious.

INGREDIENTS | SERVES 4

2 medium eggplants, peeled, cut into 16 round slices (8 each), and salted

1 cup rice or corn flour

Freshly ground black pepper, to taste

¼ cup olive oil, or as needed

Nonstick cooking spray, as needed

2 cups tomato sauce

1 pound ricotta cheese

1 cup grated Parmesan cheese, divided

2 large eggs

1 tablespoon dried oregano

1 cup shredded mozzarella cheese

Smaller Is Sweeter

The smaller eggplants now available are much sweeter and not old enough to have grown bitter. Also, many have few seeds. They come in pale cream, lavender, and purple, all the way from egg-sized to long and skinny. All are good!

1. Stack salted eggplant slices on a plate and put another plate with a weight on top to press the brown liquid out of them.

2. On a shallow plate, mix together flour and pepper. Dredge eggplant slices in flour.

3. Heat olive oil in a large skillet over medium-high heat and fry the eggplant slices until browned. Transfer to paper towels to drain.

4. Preheat oven to 325°F. Prepare a 2-quart casserole dish or a 10" × 10" glass pan with nonstick spray and spread with a thin layer of tomato sauce.

5. In a large bowl, mix together ricotta cheese, ½ cup Parmesan, eggs, and oregano. Place 1 tablespoon of the cheese mixture on each slice of eggplant and roll, placing seam-side down in the prepared baking dish.

6. Cover with remaining tomato sauce; sprinkle with remaining Parmesan and mozzarella. Bake for 35 minutes.

Chicken Divan

This is so exquisite that you won't miss potatoes, pie crust, or pasta. It stands alone as a one-dish meal.

INGREDIENTS | SERVES 6

Nonstick cooking spray, as needed

1 pound broccoli florets, cut into bite-sized pieces, cooked, and drained

3 pounds boneless, skinless chicken breasts, cut into strips

1 cup corn flour

1 teaspoon salt

Ground black pepper, to taste

½ cup olive oil, or more as needed

1½ cups Hollandaise Sauce (see recipe in this chapter)

2 tablespoons grated Parmesan cheese

Sprinkle of paprika (optional)

1. Preheat oven to 350°F. Grease a 2-quart casserole dish with nonstick spray. Make sure the cooked broccoli is well drained. You can cook it in advance and place it in the refrigerator on paper towels.

2. Roll chicken in flour, and sprinkle with salt and pepper.

3. Heat olive oil in a large sauté pan. Sauté chicken until golden brown, about 5 minutes on each side; add more oil if the pan gets dry.

4. Place the broccoli in the bottom and spoon some Hollandaise over the top. Arrange the chicken over the broccoli and pour in the rest of the sauce. Sprinkle with Parmesan cheese and paprika. Bake for 30 minutes.

Spicy Mixed Meatballs

Most meatballs have some type of bread as a filler. This recipe uses ground potato chips. The eggs will hold the balls together, and the ground chips taste wonderful.

INGREDIENTS | SERVES 4

1 pound meatloaf mix—beef, pork, and veal

2 large eggs

2 cloves garlic, minced

1 teaspoon dried oregano

½ teaspoon ground cinnamon

½ teaspoon fennel seed

½ cup finely grated Parmesan cheese

Salt and ground black pepper, to taste

2 cups crushed low-salt potato chips, divided

2 tablespoons light oil, such as canola

1. In a large bowl, mix together all ingredients except 1 cup of chips and the cooking oil. Form into meatballs about 1½–2" in diameter.

2. Place a large sheet of waxed paper on the counter. Sprinkle remaining cup of chip crumbs on it. Roll meatballs in crumbs.

3. Add oil to a large frying pan over medium-high heat. Fry meatballs until well browned on all sides. Drain on paper towels. Refrigerate, freeze, or serve immediately with the marinara sauce of your choice.

Spicy Meatballs

You can add flavor to your meatballs by grinding up some sweet or hot Italian sausage and mixing it with the beef. A truly great Italian sausage has aromatics, like garlic, herbs, and spices, such as anise seed.

Hollandaise Sauce

This sauce can be varied enormously. It's perfect on fish, lobster, or hot vegetables, especially asparagus, artichokes, and broccoli.

INGREDIENTS | MAKES 1¼ CUPS

1 cup unsalted butter

1 whole large egg

1–2 egg yolks, depending on the richness desired

1 tablespoon freshly squeezed lemon juice

⅛ teaspoon ground cayenne pepper

Salt, to taste

Hollandaise Sauce

Hollandaise sauce, with its rich, smooth texture, isn't just for eggs Benedict. It's delicious on most green vegetables, and it also pairs well with many meats and even some types of fish.

1. Melt butter in a small, heavy saucepan over very low heat. Combine egg yolks, lemon juice, and cayenne in a blender or food processor. Blend well.

2. With the motor running on low, add the hot butter, a little at a time, to the egg mixture.

3. Return the mixture to the pan you used to melt the butter. Whisking, thicken the sauce over low heat, adding salt. As soon as the sauce is thick, pour into a bowl, a sauce boat, or over the food. (Reheating the sauce to thicken it is the delicate stage. You must not let it get too hot or it will scramble the eggs, or even curdle them. If either disaster happens, add a tablespoon of boiling water and whisk like mad.)

CHAPTER 10

Vegetables, Legumes, and Sides

Lentils with Stewed Vegetables

This can be served as a main course alongside roasted cauliflower and brown rice, or as a flavorful side.

INGREDIENTS | SERVES 4

¼ cup olive oil

1 medium onion, chopped

1" piece gingerroot, peeled and coarsely chopped

5 cloves garlic, chopped

5 cups water, divided

1½ teaspoons gluten-free curry powder

½ teaspoon ground turmeric

½ teaspoon ground cumin

1 cup green lentils

2 medium carrots, quartered lengthwise, then sliced crosswise

¼ teaspoon crushed red pepper flakes

1 teaspoon salt

1 cup green peas

4 cups fresh spinach

1. Place olive oil in large pot over medium heat. Cook onion, stirring occasionally, until golden brown, about 5–7 minutes.

2. In a blender, purée ginger, garlic, and ⅓ cup water. Add purée to cooked onion and continue cooking and stirring until all water is evaporated, about 5 minutes.

3. Turn heat down to low and add curry powder, turmeric, and cumin. Stir in lentils and remaining water; simmer, covered, stirring occasionally, for about 30 minutes.

4. Add carrots, red pepper flakes, and salt; simmer, covered, stirring occasionally, until carrots are tender, about 15 minutes.

5. Stir in peas and spinach and simmer, uncovered, about 20 minutes.

Roasted Green Beans with Almonds

Dress up your everyday green beans with toasted almonds, crispy prosciutto, and fresh sage.

INGREDIENTS | SERVES 6

2 pounds green beans, trimmed

Nonstick cooking spray, as needed

2 ounces prosciutto or bacon, thinly sliced

2 teaspoons olive oil

4 cloves garlic, minced

2 teaspoons fresh sage, minced

¼ teaspoon salt, divided

Freshly ground black pepper, to taste

¼ cup almonds, toasted

1 teaspoon grated lemon zest

Toasting Nuts and Seeds

Place nuts or seeds in a dry skillet over medium-low heat and cook for 3–5 minutes. Stir gently. Your nose will know when the nuts are ready; they will have a nutty scent and will be slightly browned.

1. Fill a large pot with water and bring to a boil. Add green beans and simmer until crisp-tender, about 4 minutes. Drain green beans and set aside.

2. Spray a large pan with cooking spray and place over medium heat. Add prosciutto and cook, stirring, until crisp. Transfer prosciutto to a paper towel to blot excess oil.

3. Add olive oil to the same pan and return to medium heat. Add green beans, garlic, sage, ⅛ teaspoon salt, and pepper to the pan. Cook until the green beans begin to brown slightly

4. Add almonds, lemon zest, and prosciutto; season with remaining salt and additional pepper to taste.

White Bean Ratatouille

This is a classic French dish of stewed vegetables, often including tomatoes and eggplant, served as an appetizer or side dish. Serving it over beans makes it a bit heartier and very satisfying.

INGREDIENTS | SERVES 2

¼ cup olive oil

2 baby eggplants, chopped

1 medium onion, sliced

2 cloves garlic, minced

1 small zucchini, chopped

2 medium tomatoes, chopped

1 teaspoon each of dried parsley, thyme, and rosemary, or 1 tablespoon fresh chopped of each

Salt and ground black pepper, to taste

1 (15-ounce) can white beans, drained and rinsed

1. Heat olive oil in a large sauté pan on medium. Sauté eggplant, onion, garlic, and zucchini for 5 minutes.

2. Add tomatoes, herbs, salt, and pepper. Cover and simmer for 10 minutes. Warm the beans and serve by pouring the vegetables over the beans.

A Provençal Delight

Ratatouille is a versatile vegetable stew that can be served hot (either alone or as a side dish), at room temperature, or even cold as an appetizer on gluten-free toast or crackers. As an appetizer, it is similar to the Italian tomato, onion, and basil dish called bruschetta.

Lentil Salad

This is a salad with a burst of protein from lentils. Serve as a side or as a main lunch course.

INGREDIENTS | SERVES 4

1 pound lentils (green, yellow, or red)

1 medium onion, chopped

½ cup red wine vinegar

Salt, to taste

1 medium carrot, peeled and diced

2 large stalks celery, chopped

2 medium tomatoes, sliced

1 cup French Dressing (see recipe in Chapter 12)

1. In a large saucepan, cover the lentils with water and add onion and wine vinegar. Bring to a boil, lower heat, and simmer until soft. Sprinkle with salt.

2. Toss with diced carrot and chopped celery and arrange tomatoes around mound of lentils. Sprinkle with French Dressing and serve warm or at room temperature.

A Note about Lentils

Like other legumes, lentils are an excellent source of dietary fiber and protein. Due to their small size, lentils cook faster than other beans and legumes. Dried lentils can keep well in the pantry for up to 1 year.

Southwestern Bean Salad

This super-simple bean salad is enough to feed a small crowd at a potluck or picnic. Serve with grilled meat hot off the barbecue and a fresh green salad.

INGREDIENTS | SERVES 8

1 pound black-eyed peas

1½ cups Italian Dressing (see recipe in Chapter 12)

1 cup white corn

2 cups diced red bell peppers

1½ cups diced onion

1 cup finely chopped green onions

½ cup finely chopped jalapeño peppers

1 tablespoon finely chopped garlic

Salt, to taste

Tabasco, to taste

1. Soak peas in enough water to cover for 6 hours or overnight. Drain well.

2. Transfer peas to a medium saucepan. Add water to cover. Place over high heat and bring to a boil. Let boil until tender, about 40 minutes; do not overcook.

3. Drain peas well. Transfer peas to a large bowl. Stir in dressing and let cool.

4. Add all remaining ingredients and mix well.

Timesaving Tip

You may substitute 2 (15-ounce) cans of black-eyed peas for 1 pound of dried peas and use your favorite bottled salad dressing to speed up the preparation time. The final result will turn out just as well.

Lentil Soup with Winter Vegetables

This is a substantial soup that will warm you up and get you through a long winter.

INGREDIENTS | SERVES 4

½ pound red or yellow lentils

4 cups Vegetable Stock (see recipe in Chapter 11)

2 cups water

2 medium parsnips, peeled and chopped

2 medium carrots, peeled and chopped

2 medium white onions, chopped

4 cloves garlic, chopped

4 small bluenose turnips, peeled and chopped

½ pound deli baked ham, cut into cubes

Put all ingredients in a large soup pot and bring to a boil. Cover and simmer for 1 hour. Serve hot.

Bean and Vegetable Chili

A steaming hot bowl of this spicy chili will satisfy meat eaters and vegetarians alike.

INGREDIENTS | SERVES 8

2 tablespoons olive oil

1 medium onion, chopped

1 medium stalk celery, chopped

1 medium green bell pepper, chopped

1 medium red bell pepper, chopped

4 cloves garlic, minced

2 tablespoons chipotles in adobo, chopped

1 tablespoon ground cumin

1 tablespoon dried oregano

1 tablespoon chili powder

1½ teaspoons salt

1 (28-ounce) can diced tomatoes

3 cups water

1½ cups canned or cooked black beans, drained

3 cups canned or cooked kidney beans, drained

½ cup sour cream

1. Heat oil in a large pot over medium heat.

2. Add onion, celery, peppers, and garlic, and cook for 10 minutes.

3. Add chipotles, cumin, oregano, chili powder, and salt. Stir ingredients together. Add tomatoes and water. Reduce heat to low and simmer, uncovered, for 45 minutes.

4. Add beans and simmer for 20 minutes more.

5. Serve with a dollop of sour cream.

Classic Italian Risotto

Risotto should be very creamy on the outside,
with just a bit of toothsome resistance on the inside of each grain of rice.

INGREDIENTS | SERVES 4

2 tablespoons butter

2 tablespoons olive oil

½ cup finely chopped sweet onion

2 medium stalks celery, finely chopped

¼ cup celery leaves, chopped

1½ cups Arborio rice

1 teaspoon salt

5 cups Chicken Broth or Vegetable Stock (see recipes in Chapter 11)

¼ cup chopped fresh flat-leaf parsley

½ teaspoon ground black pepper

⅔ cup grated Parmesan cheese

1. Add butter and oil to a heavy-bottomed pot over medium heat. Melt butter, and add onion, celery, and celery leaves. Cook for 3–5 minutes, until vegetables are softened.

2. Add rice and stir to coat with butter and oil. Stir in salt. Add rice and softened vegetables to a greased 4-quart slow cooker.

3. Add remaining ingredients, except cheese, to slow cooker. Cover and cook on high for 3 hours or on low for 6 hours.

4. Stir in Parmesan cheese 20 minutes before serving.

Caramelized Onions

Caramelized onions are a great addition to roasts, dips, and sandwiches.

INGREDIENTS | MAKES 1 QUART

4 pounds Vidalia or other sweet onions

3 tablespoons butter

1 tablespoon gluten-free balsamic vinegar

Storing Caramelized Onions

Store the onions in an airtight container. They will keep up to 2 weeks refrigerated or up to 6 months frozen. If frozen, defrost overnight in the refrigerator before using.

1. Peel and slice onions into ¼" slices. Separate into rings. Thinly slice butter.

2. Place onions in a 4-quart slow cooker. Scatter butter slices over the top and drizzle with balsamic vinegar. At this point, the slow cooker may look full but the onions will quickly reduce. Cover and cook on low for 10 hours.

3. If after 10 hours the onions are wet, turn the slow cooker up to high and cook uncovered for an additional 30 minutes or until the liquid evaporates.

Baked Stuffed Artichokes

These are worth a bit of effort. You can make them in advance, then bake them just before serving.

INGREDIENTS | SERVES 4

2 large artichokes

2 tablespoons olive oil

2 cloves garlic, chopped

½ sweet onion, chopped

1 cup gluten-free cracker crumbs

1 tablespoon grated lemon zest

8 medium shrimp, peeled and deveined

¼ cup chopped fresh flat-leaf parsley

½ teaspoon ground black pepper, or to taste

4 quarts plus ½ cup water

Juice and rind of ½ lemon

½ teaspoon ground coriander

1 tablespoon grated Parmesan cheese

1. Remove any tough or brown outside leaves from artichokes. Use a sharp knife to cut off artichoke tops, about ½" down. Slam artichokes against a countertop to loosen leaves. Cut in half, from top to stem, and set aside.

2. Heat olive oil in a large frying pan over medium heat. Add garlic and onion and sauté for 5 minutes, stirring. Add cracker crumbs, lemon zest, shrimp, parsley, and pepper. Cook until shrimp turns pink. Remove from heat and pulse in a food processor or blender.

3. Boil artichokes in 4 quarts water with lemon juice, lemon rind, and coriander for 18 minutes. Reserve cooking liquid.

4. Place artichokes in a medium baking dish with ½ cup water on the bottom. Pile with shrimp filling. Drizzle with a bit of the reserved cooking liquid and sprinkle with Parmesan cheese. Bake for 25 minutes.

Garlic and Cheddar Biscuits

These cheesy morsels will remind you of the famous "Cheddar Bay" biscuits served at a popular seafood chain restaurant. For your next special dinner make a double batch to serve to guests.

INGREDIENTS | SERVES 6

1¼ cups gluten-free biscuit mix

3 tablespoons butter or Spectrum Organic All Vegetable Shortening

1 large egg

2–4 tablespoons cold water, as needed

½ cup shredded Cheddar cheese

2 cloves garlic, crushed

1. Preheat oven to 350°F. Line a baking sheet with parchment paper.

2. In a medium bowl, cut butter or shortening into biscuit mix with a fork and knife or a pastry blender until it's fully incorporated. Stir in egg and 1 tablespoon water at a time until you have a stiff but workable dough. You may not need all 4 tablespoons of water. Fold the cheese and garlic into the dough.

3. Drop 2–3 tablespoons of dough per biscuit onto prepared baking sheet about 2" apart. Gently shape each biscuit into a circle. Bake for 12–15 minutes, until golden brown. You can add a thin slice of butter on top of each biscuit and broil for about 1 minute to enhance browning. Serve hot with butter or coconut oil.

Sweet Corn Bread

This sweet corn bread is a great accompaniment to a hearty pot of chili. For extra texture and flavor add ½ cup cooked and drained sweet corn kernels and 4 slices cooked and crumbled bacon to the batter before baking.

INGREDIENTS | SERVES 6

⅓ cup brown rice flour

⅔ cup arrowroot starch

⅔ cup gluten-free cornmeal

1 teaspoon xanthan gum

2 teaspoons baking powder

½ teaspoon salt

3 tablespoons granulated sugar

¼ cup oil

2 large eggs

1 cup milk

1. Preheat oven to 425°F.

2. In a large bowl whisk together brown rice flour, arrowroot starch, and cornmeal. Add xanthan gum, baking powder, salt, and sugar. Mix thoroughly. In a smaller bowl mix together oil, eggs, and milk.

3. Mix wet ingredients into dry ingredients with a fork until you have a thick batter. Grease a 9" cake pan or iron skillet and pour batter into the pan. Spread the batter evenly over the whole pan.

4. Bake corn bread for 18–20 minutes, until golden brown and crispy around the edges. Cool for 5–10 minutes before slicing and serving.

Gluten-Free Corn Bread Stuffing

Crumble 1 recipe of day-old gluten-free corn bread. Combine in a large bowl with 1½ teaspoons poultry seasoning, 1 cup each sautéed celery and onions, and ½ teaspoon each salt and pepper. Stir in 1–2 cups gluten-free chicken broth and ¼ cup melted butter. Bake in a large casserole dish at 350°F for 20–30 minutes until the top of the stuffing is as crispy as you like it. Cool for 5 minutes before serving.

Snow Peas with Water Chestnuts and Ginger

This tasty side dish is quick, and it's good with many Asian dishes.
It's a boon to the busy working person who wants fresh vegetables but has little time.

INGREDIENTS | SERVES 4

½ cup peanut oil

1 pound snow peas, ends trimmed

1 (8-ounce) can water chestnuts, drained, rinsed, and sliced

½ cup unsalted peanuts

2 tablespoons gluten-free soy sauce

1 teaspoon lemon juice

1 tablespoon minced gingerroot

Tabasco or other red pepper sauce, to taste

1. Heat oil on high in a hot wok or frying pan and add snow peas. Stir to coat, then add water chestnuts and peanuts, stirring again. Stir-fry for 5 minutes.

2. Add remaining ingredients and mix well. Serve hot or at room temperature.

Cheese and Milk in Asian Cooking

The reason that cheese and milk are practically nonexistent in Asian cooking is that Asian countries do not have many dairy cows. In some areas, water buffalo work hard and produce milk too. Water buffalo in Italy provide the milk for a wonderful mozzarella cheese. Asians often substitute tofu for meat, and what meat they do eat is stretched with vegetables and rice. Fish is popular in lake and seaside communities. Americans have adapted Asian flavors in a popular fusion food.

Pesto with Basil and Mint

This variation on an old classic is savory with hard-boiled or poached eggs, over pasta, or as a condiment with cold meat or poultry. It's also delicious over sliced cold chicken.

INGREDIENTS | SERVES 4

½ cup pine nuts, toasted

2 cloves garlic, peeled

4 packed cups fresh basil leaves, rinsed

½ packed cup fresh mint leaves, rinsed

1 cup olive oil

1 cup grated Parmesan cheese

Salt and ground black pepper, to taste

Combine all ingredients in a food processor or blender and process until smooth. Serve as a side dish over pasta or with cold meat.

Sweet and Hot!

Mixing sweet things with a bit of spicy heat makes an intriguing flavor combo. Think of all the salsas that mix fruit with jalapeño (or even hotter) peppers—they are wonderful. Try different kinds of fruit sauces, adding a trace of peppery heat each time, until you find several you really like to serve. Experiment with mangoes, pineapple, nectarines, apricots, and whatever else is in season.

Napa Cabbage with Sesame

Napa cabbage, also called Chinese cabbage, is wonderful cooked or served raw in salads.

INGREDIENTS | SERVES 4

2 tablespoons sesame oil

2 tablespoons canola or other light oil

1 tablespoon sesame seeds

1½ pounds napa cabbage, thinly sliced

Juice of ½ lemon

2 cloves garlic, minced

Salt and ground black pepper, to taste

Gluten-free soy sauce, to taste

1. Heat oils on medium-high in a hot wok or frying pan. Add sesame seeds and toast for 2 minutes.

2. Stir in cabbage, lemon juice, and garlic. Toss until just wilted, about 4 minutes. Add salt, pepper, and soy sauce, and serve.

Apple, Cranberry, and Walnut Chutney

This is excellent with duck, chicken, and, of course, turkey. It's easy to make and will keep for 2 weeks in the refrigerator. Or make a lot and freeze it.

INGREDIENTS | MAKES 2 CUPS

½ cup finely chopped shallots

2 tablespoons canola oil

2 cups cranberries, fresh or frozen, washed and picked over if fresh

2 medium tart apples, peeled, cored, and chopped

½ cup brown sugar, or to taste

¼ cup apple cider vinegar

¼ cup water

1 teaspoon grated orange zest

½ teaspoon ground coriander seed

½ teaspoon ground black pepper

½ teaspoon salt

½ cup walnut pieces, toasted

1. In a large, heavy saucepan over medium heat, cook shallots in oil until softened.

2. Mix everything except the walnuts in with the shallots. Cook, stirring, until the cranberries have popped and the sauce has become very thick.

3. Let cool and stir in toasted walnut pieces. Store in the refrigerator.

Fruit and Pepper

Try putting some pepper on watermelon, cantaloupe, or honeydew melon. You'll find that peppery chutneys and salsas make an excellent accompaniment to all kinds of dishes.

Baked Mushroom and Fontina Risotto

You can add so many other ingredients to this risotto dish—cut-up cooked chicken or turkey, chopped pears or apples, and your favorite herbs.

INGREDIENTS | SERVES 6–8

3 tablespoons butter, divided

3 tablespoons olive oil

1 small onion, minced

2 cloves garlic, minced

Salt and ground black pepper, to taste

6 large leaves fresh sage, ripped or cut up, or 2 teaspoons dried sage, crumbled

1 cup long-grain rice

2½ cups Chicken Broth (see recipe in Chapter 11)

½ cup white vermouth

8 ounces mixed mushrooms (shiitakes, porcinis, morels, chanterelles)

⅓ cup grated fontina cheese

1. Preheat oven to 350°F.

2. Heat 1 tablespoon butter and olive oil in an ovenproof pan with a lid. Sauté onion and garlic over a low heat until softened.

3. Add salt, pepper, sage, and rice; stir to coat. Add broth and vermouth. Cover the pan and place in the oven. Bake for 20 minutes.

4. Meanwhile, melt remaining butter in a small pan over medium heat. Add mushrooms and sauté about 3–5 minutes, until well coated with butter and slightly tender.

5. Remove the pan from the oven and stir in the sautéed mushrooms. Cover the pan and continue to bake for 15 minutes.

6. Just before serving, stir in the fontina cheese.

A Misunderstood Italian Staple

Most cooks think that risotto is simply rice that has been boiled with broth and herbs. But it's so much more—the technique is simple but demanding. The secret is the rice and how it's slow cooked, using a bit of liquid until it's absorbed and then a bit more. It's been said that the rice will tell you when to add liquid—it hisses and sizzles, asking for the broth!

CHAPTER 11

Soups, Stews, and Stocks

Egg Drop Soup with Ginger and Lemon

This is a lovely spicy version of the Chinese staple, made with a variety of Asian sauces. Fish sauce is a liquid made from salted fish that is used in place of salt in many Asian recipes. Hoisin sauce is made from crushed soybeans and garlic, has a sweet and spicy flavor, and is a rich brown color.

INGREDIENTS | SERVES 2

1 tablespoon peanut oil

1 clove garlic, minced

2 cups Chicken Broth (see recipe in this chapter)

Juice of ½ lemon

1 tablespoon hoisin sauce

1 teaspoon gluten-free soy sauce

1 teaspoon fish sauce

½ teaspoon chili oil, or to taste

1" piece gingerroot, peeled and minced

2 large eggs

1. Heat peanut oil in a large saucepan. Sauté garlic over medium heat until softened, about 5 minutes.

2. Add broth, lemon juice, hoisin sauce, soy sauce, fish sauce, chili oil, and gingerroot. Stir and cover. Cook over low heat for 20 minutes.

3. Just before serving, whisk eggs with a fork. Add to the boiling soup and continue to whisk until the eggs form thin strands.

Savory Fish Stew

This stew is fresh and easy with a whole lot of flavor. The recipe calls for halibut, but just about any meaty white fish will do.

INGREDIENTS | SERVES 6

1 tablespoon olive oil

1 medium onion, finely chopped

½ cup dry white wine

3 large tomatoes, chopped

2 cups Chicken Broth (see recipe in this chapter)

1 cup clam juice

3 cups fresh spinach

1 pound halibut fillets, cut into 1" pieces

Ground white pepper, to taste

1 tablespoon chopped fresh cilantro

1. Place a large pan over medium heat. Add oil to the pan and sauté onions for 2–3 minutes. Add wine to deglaze the pan. Scrape the pan to loosen small bits of onion.

2. Add tomatoes and cook for 3–4 minutes, then add broth and clam juice to the pan. Stir in spinach and allow to wilt while continuing to stir.

3. Season fish with pepper. Place fish in the pan and cook for 5–6 minutes, until opaque. Mix in cilantro before serving.

Yellow Pepper and Tomato Soup with Basil

Yellow peppers and yellow tomatoes are very sweet and make a wonderful soup.

INGREDIENTS | SERVES 4

¼ cup peanut oil

½ cup chopped sweet white onion

2 cloves garlic, minced

1 medium yellow bell pepper, finely chopped

1½ cups Chicken Broth (see recipe in this chapter)

4 medium yellow tomatoes, cored and puréed

½ teaspoon ground cumin

½ teaspoon ground coriander

Juice of ½ lemon

Salt and ground black pepper, to taste

Fresh basil leaves, torn, for garnish

1. In a stockpot, heat oil over medium heat and sauté onion, garlic, and yellow pepper for 5 minutes. Add broth and tomatoes.

2. Stir in cumin, coriander, lemon juice, salt, and pepper. Cover and simmer for 10–15 minutes.

3. You can purée the soup if you wish or leave some bits of texture in it. Serve hot or cold and sprinkle with basil.

Colorful Veggies

Yellow fruit and vegetables are loaded with vitamin A, or retinol, which keeps your skin moist and helps your eyes adjust to changes in light. It is important to eat a variety of different colored fruit and vegetables every day.

Spiced Pumpkin Soup

If you have a sweet tooth, you can add some more brown sugar to this recipe.

INGREDIENTS | SERVES 4

1 cup finely chopped Vidalia or other sweet onion

½" piece fresh gingerroot, peeled and minced

2 cups orange juice

2 cups Chicken Broth (see recipe in this chapter)

1 (15-ounce) can pumpkin (unflavored)

1 teaspoon brown sugar

½ teaspoon ground cinnamon

¼ teaspoon ground nutmeg

¼ teaspoon ground cloves

½ cup heavy cream (optional)

Stir all ingredients into a medium soup pot one at a time, whisking after each addition. Cover and simmer for 10 minutes. If you decide to use the cream, add at the last minute.

Broccoli Soup with Cheddar

*There is a lot to love about broccoli soup. Both nourishing and full of fiber,
it can be enriched with cream or heated up with spicy pepper jack cheese.*

INGREDIENTS | SERVES 4

¼ cup olive oil

1 medium sweet onion, chopped

2 cloves garlic, chopped

1 large baking potato, peeled and
chopped

1 large bunch broccoli, coarsely
chopped

½ cup dry white wine

3 cups Chicken Broth (see recipe in this
chapter)

Salt and ground black pepper, to taste

Pinch ground nutmeg

4 heaping tablespoons grated extra-
sharp Cheddar, for garnish

1. Heat olive oil in a large stockpot. Sauté onion, garlic, and potato over medium heat until softened slightly. Add broccoli, liquids, and seasonings.

2. Cover and simmer over low heat for 45 minutes.

3. Let cool slightly. Purée in a blender. Reheat and place in bowls.

4. Spoon cheese over the hot soup to serve.

Save the Stalks

When you prepare broccoli, save the stems. They can be grated and mixed with carrots in a slaw, cut into coins and served hot, or cooked and puréed as a side. Broccoli marries well with potatoes and carrots and is good served raw with a dipping sauce.

Spinach, Sausage, and Bean Soup

This is a hearty and delicious soup. If you don't want to work with fresh spinach, get a package of frozen, chopped spinach. You can also substitute escarole or kale. Some sausage is so lean that you will need to add a bit of oil when you cook it.

INGREDIENTS | SERVES 4

1 large bunch fresh spinach, kale, or escarole, or 1 (10-ounce) package frozen, chopped spinach

8 ounces Italian sweet sausage, cut in bite-sized chunks

2 cups water, divided

2 tablespoons olive oil, or as needed

2 medium white onions, chopped

4 cloves garlic, chopped

2 medium stalks celery, chopped, leaves included

2 cups Beef Broth (see recipe in this chapter)

1 teaspoon dried oregano

1 teaspoon crushed red pepper flakes

1 (15-ounce) can red kidney beans, drained

Salt, to taste

Grated Parmesan cheese, to taste

1. Wash greens to remove any remaining grit. Stem the larger pieces and discard the thick, woody stems.

2. Place sausage in a large stockpot. Add ¾ cup water and bring to a boil; let water boil off. Add oil if dry and sauté onions, garlic, and celery for 10 minutes over medium-low heat.

3. Stir in remaining ingredients except the cheese. Cover and simmer for 35 minutes. Serve in heated bowls. Garnish with grated Parmesan cheese.

Vegetarian Option

This recipe can easily be transformed into a vegetarian-friendly soup. Substitute vegetarian sausage for Italian sausage and use vegetable broth instead of beef broth.

Beef and Sweet Potato Stew

This rich, deeply flavored beef stew with sweet potatoes, red wine, and cremini mushrooms is a crowd pleaser. Serve it over rice to absorb the delicious sauce.

INGREDIENTS | SERVES 8

¾ cup brown rice flour

1½ teaspoons salt, divided

1½ teaspoons ground black pepper, divided

1¼ pounds stew beef, cut into 1" chunks

¼ cup olive oil, divided

1 medium yellow onion, diced

2 cups peeled and diced carrots

¾ pound cremini mushrooms, cleaned and cut in half

6 cloves garlic, minced

3 tablespoons tomato paste

½ cup dry red wine

1 pound sweet potatoes, peeled and diced

4 cups Beef Broth (see recipe in this chapter)

1 dried bay leaf

1½ teaspoons dried thyme

1 tablespoon gluten-free Worcestershire sauce

1 tablespoon granulated sugar

1. In a large resealable plastic bag, combine flour, 1 teaspoon salt, and 1 teaspoon pepper. Add beef and close the bag. Shake lightly, making sure that all the beef is coated in flour and seasoning. Set aside.

2. In a large skillet, heat 2 tablespoons olive oil over medium heat. Cook beef in small batches until browned on all sides, about 1 minute per side. Add beef to a greased 4–6-quart slow cooker.

3. In the same skillet, heat remaining 2 tablespoons olive oil. Add onion and carrots and cook until onions are translucent, about 5 minutes.

4. Add mushrooms and garlic, and cook for another 2–3 minutes.

5. Add tomato paste and heat through. Deglaze the pan with the wine, scraping the stuck-on bits from the bottom of the pan. Add cooked vegetable mixture on top of beef in slow cooker.

6. Add sweet potatoes, broth, bay leaf, thyme, and Worcestershire sauce. Cover and cook on low for 8 hours or on high for 4 hours.

7. Before serving, remove bay leaf and add sugar and remaining salt and pepper.

Chicken Broth

When you remove the meat from the bones, save the dark meat for use in a casserole and the white meat for chicken salad. (To keep the chicken moist, return it to the strained broth and let it cool overnight in the refrigerator before you chop it for the salad.)

INGREDIENTS | MAKES 4 CUPS

3 pounds bone-in chicken pieces

1 large onion, peeled and quartered

2 large carrots, scrubbed

2 medium stalks celery

1 teaspoon salt

½ teaspoon ground black pepper

4½ cups water

Schmaltz

The chicken fat that will rise to the top of the broth and harden overnight in the refrigerator is known as schmaltz. You can save that fat and use it instead of butter for sautéing vegetables.

1. Add chicken pieces and onion to a 4–6-quart slow cooker.

2. Cut carrots and celery into pieces that will fit in the slow cooker, and add them to the cooker. Add salt, pepper, and water. Cover and cook on low for 6–8 hours. (Cooking time will depend on the size of the chicken pieces.) Allow to cool to room temperature.

3. Strain, discarding the cooked vegetables. Remove any meat from the chicken bones and save for another use. Refrigerate the (cooled) broth overnight. Remove and discard the hardened fat. The resulting concentrated broth can be kept for 1 week in the refrigerator or frozen for up to 3 months.

Beef Broth

Unlike chicken or turkey broth, beef broth requires a larger ratio of meat to the amount of bones used to make it. This method makes a concentrated broth. As a general rule, for regular beef broth you can usually mix ½ cup of this broth with ½ cup water.

INGREDIENTS | MAKES ABOUT 4 CUPS

1 (2-pound) bone-in chuck roast
1 pound beef bones
1 large onion, peeled and quartered
2 large carrots, scrubbed
2 medium stalks celery
1 teaspoon salt
½ teaspoon ground black pepper
4½ cups water

Boiling Broth

You don't want to let broth come to a boil during the initial cooking process because fat will render from the meat, incorporate into the broth, and make it cloudy. However, after you have strained the broth and removed the fat, you can keep it in the refrigerator longer if you bring it to a boil every other day; cool it and return it to the refrigerator until needed.

1. Add chuck roast, beef bones, and onion to a 4-quart or larger slow cooker. Cut carrots and celery into pieces that will fit in the slow cooker, and add them to the cooker. Add salt, pepper, and water. Cover and cook on low for 8 hours.

2. Use a slotted spoon to remove the roast and beef bones. Reserve the meat removed from the bones for another use; discard the bones.

3. Once the broth has cooled enough to make it easier to handle, strain it; discard the cooked vegetables. Refrigerate the (cooled) broth overnight. Remove and discard the hardened fat. The resulting concentrated broth can be kept for 1 week in the refrigerator or frozen for up to 3 months.

Vegetable Stock

This is a great recipe for using up leftover vegetables and peelings. Vegetable stock is a healthy ingredient to keep in the fridge to make quick soups or to cook gluten-free starches such as rice and potatoes.

INGREDIENTS | MAKES ABOUT 6 CUPS

2 medium carrots, peeled and roughly chopped

1 large onion, quartered

3 cloves garlic

2 medium stalks celery, roughly chopped

2 red potatoes, quartered (peeled or unpeeled)

6 cups water

1 teaspoon salt

1 teaspoon ground black pepper

1. Place chopped vegetables in a 4–6-quart slow cooker.

2. Pour water over the vegetables and add salt and pepper.

3. Cover and cook on high for 4–6 hours or on low for 8–10 hours.

4. Allow broth to cool slightly and then strain out and discard vegetables. Pour stock into clean glass jars and refrigerate for up to 1 week or freeze for several months until needed. If you plan to freeze the stock either store in resealable plastic bags or leave 2" of room in each glass jar to allow liquids to expand.

Reducing Stocks

A simple way to add more flavor to your stock is to simply cook it down (reduce it by half) in a pot on the stove. Reduced stocks have a great depth of flavor and can be used as a sauce, gravy, or as the liquid to cook rice, potatoes, or gluten-free pasta.

Fish Stock

Use fish stock in any fish or seafood dish instead of water or chicken stock.

INGREDIENTS | MAKES 3 QUARTS

3 quarts water

2 medium onions, quartered

Head and bones from 3 whole fish, any type

2 medium stalks celery, chopped

2 tablespoons peppercorns

1 bunch fresh flat-leaf parsley

1. Place all ingredients into a 4–6-quart slow cooker. Cook on low for 8–10 hours.

2. Strain out all the solids. Refrigerate overnight. The next day skim off any foam that has floated to the top. You can use the stock immediately or refrigerate or freeze it for later use. Stock will stay fresh in the fridge for up to 1 week and up to 6 months in the freezer.

Hearty Lamb Stew

Make a double recipe and freeze half for another busy day.
You can cook beans the old-fashioned way, or use canned cannellini beans instead.

INGREDIENTS | SERVES 6

¼ cup olive oil

2 pounds lamb stew meat

½ cup potato flour

Salt and ground black pepper, to taste

2 slices bacon, chopped

4 cloves garlic, chopped

2 large onions, chopped

2 medium carrots, peeled and chopped

2 dried bay leaves

2 cups Chicken Broth (see recipe in this chapter)

1 cup dry white wine

½ bunch fresh flat-leaf parsley

2 tablespoons dried rosemary

Juice and zest of ½ lemon

2 teaspoons gluten-free Worcestershire sauce

3 (15-ounce) cans white beans, drained

1. Heat olive oil in a large, heavy-bottomed stew pot. Dredge lamb in flour mixed with salt and pepper. Add meat and bacon to pot and cook until browned. Add garlic, onions, carrots, and bay leaves, and cook until soft.

2. Add broth, wine, and herbs. Stir in lemon juice and zest and Worcestershire sauce.

3. Cover and cook for 3 hours. Pour off broth and put in the freezer to bring the fat to the top. When the meat is cool enough to handle, remove from the bones.

4. Return the meat and broth to the pot. If too thin, mix 2 tablespoons cornstarch with 3 tablespoons water, add, and bring to a boil.

5. Stir in beans. Cover and simmer for 20 minutes. Remove bay leaf before serving.

Using Dried Beans

If you'd rather use dried beans instead of the canned in this stew it's an easy switch. Just take 1 pound great northern beans and soak them overnight. The next day, drain the beans and simmer them in fresh water for 5 hours. Then the beans are ready to be added to the stew.

New England Clam Chowder

This recipe is very traditional. Many cooks now substitute bacon for salt pork, but it's better to make it the traditional way.

INGREDIENTS | SERVES 4

2 dozen cherrystone clams (2" across)

2 cups water

3 ounces salt pork, finely chopped

1 large onion, chopped

1 medium carrot, peeled and chopped

2 medium stalks celery with tops, finely chopped

2 large Idaho potatoes, peeled and chopped

1–2 tablespoons cornstarch (depending on how thick you like your chowder)

2 dried bay leaves

1 teaspoon dried thyme

1 teaspoon celery salt

1 tablespoon Worcestershire sauce

3 cups clam broth

1 cup whole milk

1 cup heavy cream

Freshly ground black pepper, to taste

½ cup chopped fresh flat-leaf parsley, for garnish

1. Scrub clams and place in a large pot. Add water, cover, and boil until the clams open. Remove them to a large bowl and let cool; reserve the juice. When cool, remove the clams, discard the shells, and chop the clams in a food processor.

2. In a soup pot, fry salt pork on medium until crisp. Drain on paper towels. Add vegetables to the soup pot and sauté over medium heat until soft, about 10 minutes. Blend in cornstarch and cook for 2 more minutes, stirring.

3. Add reserved clam juice, bay leaves, thyme, and celery salt. Stir in Worcestershire sauce, clam broth, chopped clams, and salt pork. Cover and simmer for ½ hour.

4. Bring to a slow boil before adding milk and cream. Reduce heat to a simmer and cover to let the ingredients marry. (After you add the milk and cream, do not boil. If you do, your soup is likely to curdle.)

5. Before serving, remove bay leaves. Add black pepper to taste. Garnish with chopped fresh parsley, and serve hot.

Is That Clam Alive or Dead?

Never eat a dead clam. Always run them under cold water and scrub vigorously with a brush. To test for life, tap two clams together. You should hear a sharp click, not a hollow thud. If the clam sounds hollow, tap it again, and then, if still hollow-sounding, discard it. If you're cooking clams in the shell, be sure to discard any unopened clams after cooking is complete. Those are dead too.

Asian-Style Soup with Rice Noodles

This can be served in small bowls as a first course or in large bowls as lunch. The contrast between soft and crunchy, spicy and sweet makes this an interesting soup.

INGREDIENTS | SERVES 4

1 quart Chicken Broth (see recipe in this chapter)

2 cloves garlic, minced

1" piece fresh gingerroot, peeled and minced

1 bunch scallions, thinly sliced

12 canned water chestnuts

1 cup bean sprouts, well rinsed

½ cup dry sherry

½ cup gluten-free soy sauce

½ pound satin tofu

2 cups rice noodles, cooked

12 snow peas, sliced on the diagonal, for garnish

1. Bring broth to a boil in a large soup pot. Add all ingredients except the tofu, noodles, and snow peas. Cover and simmer for 10 minutes. Add tofu.

2. Stir gently and add cooked noodles. Garnish with snow peas and serve.

Soy Galore

Tofu is made of soy and is related to all soy products, such as soy sauce, soy nuts, and soy paste. All are excellent food supplements. Tofu comes in satin (very soft and custardy), medium, firm, and extra-firm. The firm is excellent fried. The more tofu you eat, the better off your arteries will be—it has no cholesterol.

Shrimp and Coconut Soup

This is equally good served chilled or hot. You can add 1 cup of cooked rice to this, but it is not necessary.

INGREDIENTS | SERVES 4

2 shallots, minced

2 teaspoons peanut oil or vegetable oil

2 tablespoons cornstarch

1½ cups Shrimp Shell Broth (see sidebar), warmed

½ cup dry white wine

1 cup unsweetened coconut milk

1 cup cooked rice (optional)

1 pound medium shrimp, shelled, deveined, and chopped

Salt and freshly ground white pepper, to taste

1. In a large saucepan over medium heat, sauté shallots in oil until soft, about 10 minutes. Stir in cornstarch and cook until very thick.

2. Add liquid ingredients and cook, covered, over low heat for 30 minutes.

3. Stir in rice (if using) and shrimp; heat until the shrimp turns pink, about 5 minutes. Add salt and white pepper to taste and serve hot or cold.

Shrimp Shell Broth

Shrimp Shell Broth makes a flavorful addition to seafood soup. Next time you are preparing shrimp, reserve the shells. Add 1 cup of water, 1 cup of wine, and 1 bay leaf to the shells from 1 pound of shrimp. Bring to a boil, lower heat, and simmer, covered, for 20 minutes. Remove bay leaf. Strain and use as broth in your soup.

Cashew-Zucchini Soup

Cashews make this soup thick and creamy and provide a serving of heart-healthy fat.

INGREDIENTS | SERVES 4

4 medium zucchini

Nonstick cooking spray, as needed

1 large Vidalia onion, chopped

4 cloves garlic, chopped

½ teaspoon salt, plus extra to taste

¼ teaspoon ground black pepper, plus extra to taste

3 cups Vegetable Stock (see recipe in this chapter)

½ cup raw cashews

½ teaspoon dried tarragon

Cashew Nut Butter

You may substitute the whole raw cashews in this recipe with cashew nut butter. You can enjoy using the leftover cashew nut butter as a spread on sandwiches and as a dip for fresh fruit. Remember when snacking on nut butters that they are high in calories, so limit your portion size.

1. Coarsely chop the 4 zucchini.

2. Spray a large saucepan with nonstick cooking spray. Add onion to the pan and cook for 5 minutes over medium heat, until soft and translucent. Add garlic and cook for 1 minute. Stir in chopped zucchini, ½ teaspoon salt, and ¼ teaspoon pepper; cook over medium heat, covered, stirring occasionally, for 5 minutes.

3. Add stock and simmer for 15 minutes.

4. Add cashews and tarragon. Purée soup in a blender in batches. Only fill blender halfway to avoid burns from the hot liquid.

5. Return soup to the pot; season with additional salt and pepper as desired.

CHAPTER 12

Salads and Dressings

Grilled Eggplant and Pepper Salad

Grill the eggplant and peppers the day before a party, then, at the last minute, put the vegetables together, shave the provolone, and dress the salad.

INGREDIENTS | SERVES 12

⅓ cup balsamic or red wine vinegar

1 cup olive oil

1 teaspoon gluten-free Dijon mustard

Salt and ground black pepper, to taste

1 medium eggplant, peeled and sliced into ½" rounds

3 medium red bell peppers, cored, seeded, and cut in half

1 large bunch arugula or watercress, stems removed

1 large head romaine lettuce, chopped

4 ripe tomatoes, cored and chopped

2 ounces aged provolone cheese

1. Prepare the dressing: Mix together the vinegar, oil, mustard, and salt and pepper in a cruet. Shake well.

2. Brush eggplant slices with some of the dressing, and grill on medium heat for 3 minutes on each side. Let cool and cut into cubes.

3. Grill the peppers skin-side down until charred. Place in a paper bag. Let cool, then peel off the skin. Cut into pieces.

4. Just before serving, toss the greens with the eggplant and peppers, add tomatoes, and shave provolone over the top.

5. Blend the remaining dressing in a blender. Pour over the salad.

BLT Salad with Turkey and Avocado

This is a satisfying lunch salad; it's delicious and easy to make. You can also put it on a gluten-free bun and serve it as a sandwich. For a lighter option, you can either omit the bacon or substitute it with vegetarian bacon or Canadian bacon.

INGREDIENTS | SERVES 4

4 strips bacon

1 pound deli turkey breast

1 pint cherry tomatoes, halved

1 large ripe avocado, peeled and diced

½ cup low-fat mayonnaise

½ cup French Dressing (see recipe in this chapter)

2 cups shredded lettuce

1. In a medium skillet, fry bacon until crisp, about 7–10 minutes. Cool on a paper towel–lined plate, then crumble into a large serving bowl.

2. Thickly dice turkey breast.

3. Combine all ingredients except lettuce in the bowl and mix well. Serve over lettuce.

Salad Dressings

Did you ever study the labels of commercial salad dressings? There are chemicals and preservatives in these dressings that you may not want to ingest. Save a jar of olive juice after you've eaten the olives. Make your own dressing and know that everything in it is healthy!

Fig and Parmesan Curl Salad

This mixture may sound a bit different, and it is! In addition to being unique, it is also delicious.

INGREDIENTS | SERVES 2

4 fresh figs, cut into halves, or 4 dried figs, plumped in 1 cup boiling water and soaked for ½ hour

2 cups fresh baby spinach, stems removed

¼ cup olive oil

Juice of ½ lemon

2 tablespoons gluten-free balsamic vinegar

1 teaspoon honey

1 teaspoon gluten-free dark brown mustard

Salt and ground black pepper, to taste

4 large curls Parmesan cheese

1. When the figs (if dried) are softened, arrange them and the spinach on serving dishes.

2. In a small bowl, whisk together olive oil, lemon juice, balsamic vinegar, honey, mustard, salt, and pepper.

3. Make Parmesan curls with a vegetable peeler and place over figs and spinach; drizzle with dressing.

A Hidden Gem

Figs are a wonderfully nutritious food. Not only are they high in fiber and minerals, but they also add tons of flavor to any recipe. Some cultures even claim that figs have medicinal value and healing potential.

Shrimp and Blood Orange Salad

For an elegant supper or luncheon salad, this is a crowd-pleaser. The deep red flesh of the blood oranges contrasted with the saturated green of spinach, and the bright pink shrimp makes for a dramatic presentation!

INGREDIENTS | SERVES 4

2 (6-ounce) bags baby spinach (try to find prewashed)

2 medium blood oranges

1¼ pounds medium shrimp, peeled, deveined, cooked, and chilled

Juice of ½ lemon

¼ cup extra-virgin olive oil

¼ teaspoon dry mustard

Salt and ground black pepper, to taste

¼ loosely packed cup stemmed parsley or cilantro

1. Place spinach on individual serving plates.

2. Peel oranges and cut into ¼"-thick slices, picking out any seeds. Arrange on top of spinach. Arrange shrimp around oranges.

3. Place remaining ingredients in a blender and purée until the dressing is bright green. Pour over the salads. Serve chilled.

Fresh Spinach—Not Lettuce

Substitute fresh baby spinach for less nutritious iceberg lettuce. White or pale green lettuce can be used as accents but have less nutritional substance than such greens as spinach, escarole, chicory, and watercress.

Spicy Asian Salad with Grilled Tuna

The fish is hot, the vegetables are spicy, and the greens are chilled!
This is an exotic salad that is deceptively easy to make.

INGREDIENTS | SERVES 4

3 tablespoons sesame oil

½ cup olive oil

2 cloves garlic, minced

1 teaspoon minced fresh gingerroot

2 teaspoons sherry vinegar

1 tablespoon gluten-free soy sauce

2–3 cups shredded napa cabbage

1 medium red onion, cut into wedges

2 Japanese eggplants, sliced lengthwise

4 (¼-pound) tuna steaks

1. In a small bowl, whisk together sesame oil, olive oil, garlic, ginger, sherry vinegar, and soy sauce. Divide into 2 portions and set aside.

2. Place cabbage on serving plates.

3. Paint onion, eggplant, and tuna with 1 portion of the dressing, being careful not to contaminate the dressing with the utensil that touched the fish.

4. Grill the vegetables and tuna for 3–4 minutes per side over medium heat. Arrange the vegetables and fish over the cabbage. Drizzle with the reserved dressing.

A Quick Meal

Tuna are large fish in the mackerel family. They have a unique circulatory system that allows them to retain a higher body temperature than the cool waters they inhabit. This provides tuna with an extra burst of energy that allows them to reach short-distance swimming speeds of over 40 miles per hour!

Fresh Gluten-Free Croutons

*These can be made in advance and stored in the refrigerator,
then crisped up at the last moment. Double the recipe for extras.*

INGREDIENTS | MAKES 24 CROUTONS

½ cup olive oil
2 cloves garlic, minced
4 thick-cut slices gluten-free bread,
 crusts removed
Salt and ground black pepper, to taste
Nonstick cooking spray, as needed

For the Love of Garlic

Garlic has various degrees of potency
depending on how you cut it. Finely
minced garlic, or that which has been put
through a press, will be the strongest.
When garlic is sliced, it is less strong, and
when you leave the cloves whole, they are
even milder.

1. Preheat broiler to 350°F.

2. Mix together oil and garlic. Brush both sides of bread
   with garlic oil. Sprinkle with salt and pepper to taste.

3. Cut each slice of bread into 6 cubes, to make 24 cubes.
   Spray a baking sheet with nonstick spray. Place the
   cubes on the sheet and broil until well browned on
   both sides.

4. Put the baking sheet on the bottom rack of the oven.
   Turn off the oven and leave the croutons to dry for 20
   minutes.

5. Store in an airtight container until ready to use.

Wild Rice Salad

This is just as good on a summer picnic as it is a wintry side dish. It's filling and delightful.

INGREDIENTS | SERVES 6

4 cups water

¾ cup wild rice

1 teaspoon salt

Ground black pepper, to taste

1 small red onion, chopped

3 medium stalks celery, chopped finely

1 cup water chestnuts, drained and chopped

1 cup jicama, peeled and chopped

1 small apple, cored and chopped

⅔ cup olive oil

⅓ cup raspberry vinegar

½ cup chopped fresh flat-leaf parsley

6 ounces fresh raspberries, rinsed and set on paper towels to dry

1. Bring water to a boil and add rice; return to a rolling boil and then reduce heat to simmer and cover tightly. After 30 minutes, add salt and pepper.

2. When the rice has bloomed but is still hot (about 40–60 minutes more), add vegetables and apple. Taste and add salt and pepper if desired.

3. Whisk together olive oil, vinegar, and parsley in a small bowl, and combine with the rice and vegetables. Place in a large serving dish and serve warm or chilled. Sprinkle with berries at the last minute.

Cooking Wild Rice

Disregard the directions on the package of wild rice. They tell you to cook for 30–40 minutes, when it takes more like 90 minutes for it to bloom and soften. When cooking, just keep adding liquid if the rice dries out, and keep simmering until it "blooms," or the grains open up.

French Dressing

This is a great dressing on a crisp green salad.
You can also use it as a marinade for beef, chicken, or pork.

INGREDIENTS | MAKES 1 CUP

⅓ cup red wine vinegar

½ teaspoon gluten-free Worcestershire sauce

1 clove garlic, chopped

2 tablespoons chopped fresh flat-leaf parsley

1 teaspoon dried thyme

1 teaspoon dried rosemary

Pinch granulated sugar

⅔ cup extra-virgin olive oil

Mix together all ingredients except olive oil in a blender. Slowly add the oil in a thin stream so that the ingredients will emulsify.

Lemon Pepper Dressing

Peppercorns and chilies offer different flavors in cooking. Peppercorns are dried berries, and chilies are the hot fruit of a plant and have spicy seeds. This recipe is a wonderful marriage of pepper flavors. Use it with grilled vegetables, as well as on salads.

INGREDIENTS | MAKES 1 CUP

7 ounces low-fat mayonnaise

Juice and zest of ½ lemon

1 teaspoon gluten-free Dijon mustard

1 teaspoon freshly ground black pepper

½ teaspoon ground white pepper

½ teaspoon crushed red pepper flakes

Salt, to taste

¼ teaspoon anchovy paste

Whisk together all ingredients and serve with chicken, salad, or cold meats.

Italian Dressing

You can find garlic paste in a tube at health food stores and online. It's a good way to get garlic flavoring throughout a dish without little bits of the vegetable.

INGREDIENTS | MAKES ½ CUP

¼ cup extra-virgin olive oil

2 tablespoons gluten-free balsamic vinegar

1 tablespoon red wine vinegar

1 teaspoon garlic paste

1 teaspoon dried basil

½ teaspoon dried oregano

2 teaspoons dried parsley flakes

¼ teaspoon salt

⅛ teaspoon ground white pepper

1. In small bowl, combine olive oil, vinegars, and garlic paste and whisk to blend and distribute garlic paste evenly.

2. Add remaining ingredients and whisk to blend. Store covered in refrigerator for up to 4 days.

Is Balsamic Vinegar Gluten-Free?

Not all balsamic vinegar is gluten-free. This vinegar gets its deep color and rich flavor from long aging in oak casks. The more inexpensive varieties may get that deep color from caramel coloring or other additives, which can contain gluten. To be safe, buy the best-quality balsamic vinegar you can afford, and be sure the ingredient label has only one ingredient: vinegar.

Caesar Dressing

True Caesar salad dressing has a touch of anchovy, lemon, and mustard.

INGREDIENTS | MAKES 1 CUP

¼ cup red wine vinegar

1 large (pasteurized) egg

1 clove garlic, mashed

1 tablespoon lemon juice

½ teaspoon dry mustard

½ teaspoon anchovy paste

Salt and ground black pepper, to taste

¼ cup grated Parmesan cheese

¼ cup extra-virgin olive oil

1. In a blender, blend vinegar, egg, garlic, and lemon juice until puréed. Add mustard, anchovy paste, salt, pepper, and cheese.

2. With the blender running on medium speed, slowly pour in the olive oil in a thin stream.

Which Olive Oil Is Best?

Extra-virgin olive oil comes from the first pressing of the olives, has the most intense flavor, and is the most expensive. Use this for salads and for dressings and dips. Virgin olive oil is from the second pressing. Less expensive than extra-virgin, it can be used for the same purposes. "Olive oil" indicates that it is from the last pressing; this is the oil used for cooking since it does not burn as easily at high temperatures.

Sweet and Sour Dressing

You can use this as a dressing for salad, especially Asian noodle salads, or hot noodles.
You can also use it on pork, chicken, or beef.

INGREDIENTS | MAKES ½ CUP

6 tablespoons gluten-free soy sauce

1 teaspoon Asian sesame oil

1 teaspoon minced fresh gingerroot

1 tablespoon maple syrup or honey

1 tablespoon concentrated orange juice

1 tablespoon apricot preserves or jam

1 clove garlic, minced

1 teaspoon Tabasco sauce, or to taste

Whisk together all ingredients in a small saucepan over low heat until well blended and serve.

Spinach Fruit Salad

This sweet and tangy salad dressing is good on any mixed greens; try it on coleslaw, too.

INGREDIENTS | SERVES 6

Dressing:
½ cup sliced strawberries
1 tablespoon lemon juice
1 tablespoon granulated sugar
¼ teaspoon salt
1 tablespoon gluten-free yellow mustard
1 tablespoon minced onion
¼ cup apple juice
¼ cup extra-virgin olive oil
Salad:
6 cups baby spinach
2 cups watercress
2 cups sliced strawberries
1 cup raspberries

1. Combine all dressing ingredients in a food processor or blender; process or blend until smooth. Cover and refrigerate up to 3 days.

2. In large serving bowl, toss together all salad ingredients. Drizzle with half of the dressing; toss again. Serve immediately with remaining dressing on the side.

Greens and Fruit Salad

This salad dressing can be used on any tossed salad. Try it the next time you make a pasta salad.

INGREDIENTS | SERVES 4

4 cups mixed salad greens

2 cups baby spinach leaves

2 cups red grapes

1 medium orange, peeled and chopped

¼ cup orange juice

2 tablespoons honey

¼ cup extra-virgin olive oil

1 tablespoon gluten-free Dijon mustard

¼ teaspoon ground ginger

¼ teaspoon salt

⅛ teaspoon ground white pepper

1. In serving bowl, toss together salad greens, spinach, grapes, and orange; set aside.

2. In a small bottle with a screw-top lid, combine remaining ingredients. Seal lid and shake vigorously to blend salad dressing. Pour over salad, toss lightly, and serve immediately.

Packaged Greens or Fresh?

For the freshest greens, pick those that have not been processed and packaged and are ready to use. There is less risk of cross-contamination, and you have control over exactly what is in your salad. Wash the greens by rinsing in cold water, then dry by rolling the leaves in a kitchen towel.

CHAPTER 13

Snacks

Spicy Guacamole

A traditional guacamole is a crowd-pleasing appetizer or a tasty addition to a simple sandwich or wrap.

INGREDIENTS | SERVES 4

2 medium ripe avocados

½ red onion, minced (about ½ cup)

2 tablespoons finely chopped cilantro leaves

Juice of 1 lime

Salt and freshly ground black pepper, to taste

1 serrano chili

½ tomato, chopped

Working with Hot Chilies

Put on rubber gloves when handling hot chili peppers. They can sting, burn, and irritate the skin. Avoid touching your eyes during or after working with chilies. Be sure to wash your hands with soap and warm water right after.

1. Cut avocados in half. Remove the seed and peel. Place in a medium mixing bowl and mash with a fork.

2. Add onion, cilantro, lime juice, salt, and pepper. Mix ingredients together.

3. Cut open chili pepper and scrape out stems, seeds, and veins with the tip of a knife. Mince the pepper and add to the guacamole to your desired degree of hotness.

4. Add chopped tomatoes just before serving.

Deviled Eggs with Capers

If deviled eggs aren't spicy, they aren't devilish enough! This recipe can be adapted if you want less heat. Deviled eggs are easy to make and transport—great for a picnic or brunch.

INGREDIENTS | SERVES 4

6 large hard-boiled eggs, shelled and cut in half

½ cup low-fat mayonnaise

1 teaspoon Tabasco

1 teaspoon celery salt

1 teaspoon onion powder

1 teaspoon garlic powder

1 chili pepper of your choice, finely minced, or to taste

2 tablespoons extra-small capers, rinsed and drained

Paprika or chopped chives, for garnish

1. Scoop out egg yolks and place in a food processor along with mayonnaise, Tabasco, celery salt, onion powder, garlic powder, chili pepper, and capers. Blend until smooth and spoon into the hollows in the eggs.

2. Garnish with paprika or chives. Chill, covered with aluminum foil tented above the egg yolk mixture.

Brine-Packed Capers

Capers are actually berries that have been pickled. You can get them packed in salt, but they are better when packed in brine. You can get larger ones or very, very small ones—the tiny ones are tastier.

Stuffed Zucchini Boats

Zucchini acts as the perfect vessel for this tempting snack. A finger food topped with cheese and marinara sauce is a sure crowd-pleaser as an appetizer, too.

INGREDIENTS | SERVES 2

2 large zucchini

1 teaspoon olive oil

Salt and ground black pepper, to taste

4 ounces ground turkey

¼ cup marinara sauce

2 ounces part-skim ricotta cheese

1 tablespoon grated Parmesan cheese

Low-Fat Option

To reduce the total calories and fat in the zucchini boats, choose low-fat or fat-free ricotta cheese. The recipe calls for ground turkey since it is leaner than ground beef. Vegetarians or those looking for a meat-free meal can substitute the ground turkey with ground soy "meat."

1. Set oven rack at upper-middle position and turn broiler to high.

2. Slice each zucchini in half lengthwise. Using a spoon, remove seeds from zucchini halves, creating a hollow center.

3. Rub zucchini with oil and season with salt and pepper to taste. Place on a baking sheet with open side facing up. Broil for 8 minutes or until zucchini are fork tender.

4. Meanwhile, brown ground turkey in a medium pan over medium heat.

5. Heat marinara sauce in a small saucepan.

6. Remove zucchini from oven and transfer to a platter.

7. Combine ground turkey and marinara sauce. Spread a thin layer of ricotta cheese across zucchini; top with meat sauce. Sprinkle with Parmesan cheese.

Brie-Stuffed Celery with Walnuts

*This unique take on stuffed celery is wonderful, replacing peanut butter
or cream cheese with luxurious, buttery Brie.*

INGREDIENTS | SERVES 6

6 large celery stalks

5 ounces Brie cheese, softened

2 tablespoons capers, rinsed and
  drained

3 tablespoons chopped walnuts, toasted

1. Trim off thin portion of celery stalks and discard. Cut remaining wide ends in half crosswise. Lay celery pieces on a cool serving plate. Remove the skin from the Brie then mash with a fork. Mix in capers.

2. Stuff each piece of celery with cheese and garnish with toasted walnuts.

Fruit Skewers with Yogurt Dip

A forkless version of the fruit salad, this appetizer can be made with a variety of seasonal fruit.

INGREDIENTS | SERVES 4

4 kiwifruit, sliced into ½" pieces

8 large strawberries, sliced in half

2 medium pears, cut into ½" pieces

1 large orange, sliced into ½" pieces

1 cup plain low-fat yogurt

Juice of 1 lime

2 teaspoons finely chopped fresh mint leaves

1. Arrange cut fruit pieces on 8 wooden skewers, alternating fruit types.

2. In a small bowl, mix together yogurt, lime juice, and mint.

3. Serve fruit skewers with yogurt dip.

Fresh Herbed Yogurt

Herbs and citrus make yogurt taste great. For a different flavor, try using fresh basil leaves and the juice of half a lemon. You can also use other low-GI fresh fruit like bananas and apples.

Black Bean Salsa

This zesty and colorful salsa may be served alone or with a spicy Southwestern dish.

INGREDIENTS | MAKES 6 CUPS

4 cups chopped tomatoes
2 cups cooked black beans
1 cup diced onion
1 jalapeño, seeded and diced
½ cup chopped fresh cilantro
Juice of 2 limes
Salt and ground black pepper, to taste

1. Mix together tomatoes, beans, onion, jalapeño, cilantro, and lime juice in a medium bowl.

2. Add salt and pepper as desired.

Mango Salsa

This is excellent with shrimp, crab legs, or fruit. Avoid using frozen mango since it tends to be mushy when thawed.

INGREDIENTS | MAKES 1 CUP

1 large mango, peeled and diced

¼ cup minced sweet onion

2 teaspoons apple cider vinegar

2 jalapeño peppers, cored, seeded, and minced

Juice of ½ lime

2 tablespoons finely chopped fresh cilantro or flat-leaf parsley

Salt, to taste

Pulse all ingredients in a food processor or blender. Turn into a bowl, chill, and serve.

Mango Facts

Did you know mangoes are the most popular fruit in the world? They are grown in tropical climates and are available to be enjoyed year round. In many countries, mango is eaten both ripe and unripe. The unripe mango is often pickled, seasoned, or made into a sauce and served with a savory meal. Sweet, ripe mangoes can be made into juice, smoothies, and fruit salads.

Tex-Mex Taco Dip

This is a super-easy gluten-free taco dip made with everyday pantry ingredients.

INGREDIENTS | SERVES 6

Nonstick cooking spray, as needed

1 (8-ounce) package cream cheese

1 (14.5-ounce) can diced tomatoes, drained, ¼ cup juice reserved

½ cup refried beans

1 (1.25-ounce) package gluten-free taco seasoning

¼ cup sliced black olives

Make Your Own Taco Seasoning

You can create your own taco seasoning to keep on hand by mixing together: 1 tablespoon chili powder, ¼ teaspoon garlic powder, ¼ teaspoon onion powder, ¼ teaspoon dried oregano, ½ teaspoon paprika, 1½ teaspoons cumin, 1 tablespoon granulated sugar, ½ teaspoon salt, and ½ teaspoon ground black pepper. Store in an airtight container and use when a recipe calls for taco seasoning.

1. Grease a 1.5-quart slow cooker with nonstick cooking spray.

2. Add cream cheese, drained diced tomatoes, reserved tomato juice, refried beans, and taco seasoning. Mix together, cover, and cook on low for 4–5 hours or on high for 2–2½ hours.

3. Right before serving, sprinkle sliced black olives on top of dip. Serve with gluten-free corn chips, rice chips, or gluten-free toast points.

Rosemary Basil Crackers or Crispy Pizza Crust

This versatile recipe can make crispy, crunchy crackers or a cracker-like pizza crust. Either is delicious and incredibly easy to make.

INGREDIENTS | MAKES 1 (12") PIZZA CRUST OR 30–40 SMALL CRACKERS

1¾ cup blanched almond flour, plus extra for rolling out dough

½ teaspoon sea salt

1 teaspoon dried, crushed rosemary

1 teaspoon dried basil

2 tablespoons olive oil

1 large egg

1. Preheat oven to 350°F.

2. In a medium mixing bowl whisk together blanched almond flour, sea salt, dried rosemary, and dried basil. Whisk together. Make a well in the center of dry ingredients and add olive oil and egg.

3. Mix egg and olive oil into the dry ingredients thoroughly until you have a stiff dough.

4. Place a 12" × 16" sheet of parchment paper on a large baking sheet. Lightly sprinkle blanched almond flour over the parchment paper and place the dough in the middle, on top of flour. Place a sheet of plastic wrap gently over the dough as a barrier between the dough and the rolling pin. Roll to ¼" thickness or roughly into a 10" × 14" rectangle. Score crackers by gently rolling a pizza cutter over the dough in a crisscross pattern to create about 30–40 (1") squares. For a pizza crust, roll into an 11" × 11" circle.

5. For crackers: bake for 12–15 minutes until crackers are lightly golden brown around the edges. Remove from oven and let cool for 20 minutes before breaking into individual crackers. Cool completely on the parchment paper and store any leftover crackers in an airtight container for up to 1 week on the counter. Baked crackers will freeze well for up to 2 months in an airtight container.

6. For pizza: par-bake crust for 10 minutes until it's just crispy. Add toppings and bake an additional 10–12 minutes until toppings have heated through. Allow to cool for 5 minutes and then cut and serve with salad.

Chili Bean Dip with Dipping Vegetables

This is a great addition to any snack tray, whether for watching a game on TV or after school. Serve with corn bread or your favorite gluten-free crackers.

INGREDIENTS | MAKES 1 QUART

½ pound ground beef

1 medium onion, chopped

2 jalapeño peppers, or to taste, cored, seeded, and chopped

2 cloves garlic, chopped

¼ cup vegetable oil

4 teaspoons chili powder, or to taste

1 (15-ounce) can crushed tomatoes with juice

1 (15-ounce) can red kidney beans

½ cup flat beer

Assortment of carrots, celery pieces, radishes, broccoli, spears of zucchini, etc.

1. In a medium sauté pan over medium heat, sauté the beef, onion, jalapeño peppers, and garlic in the oil, breaking up the meat with a spoon to avoid clumping.

2. When the vegetables are soft, add the remaining ingredients (except the vegetables for dipping). Cover and simmer for 1 hour.

3. Serve warm. Or cool, and turn this into a dip by pulsing it in a food processor. Do not make it smooth. Serve alongside veggies.

Chili and Beans

There are endless variations of the chili-and-bean combination. Some people use turkey, others add dark chocolate and cinnamon and vary the amounts of beans and tomatoes. Some forms of chili don't have any beans. Various regions use various amounts of spice, heat, and ingredients.

Tomatillo Salsa

Tomatillos are small green tomato-like fruit with papery husks.
They are available in many supermarkets and all Latino markets.

INGREDIENTS | MAKES ABOUT 1 CUP

10–12 tomatillos, husked, rinsed, and chopped

2 tablespoons olive oil

1 medium yellow tomato, cored and finely chopped

½ red onion, finely chopped

2 cloves garlic, minced

Juice of 1 lime and ½ teaspoon lime zest

2 serrano chilies, cored, seeded, and minced

1 teaspoon salt, or to taste

¼ cup minced fresh flat-leaf parsley or cilantro

Combine all ingredients in a bowl and cover. Let stand for 2 hours or refrigerate overnight. Serve at room temperature.

Tropical Fruit Salsa

The sweet-hot combination of this salsa is wonderful. Try it with pork, lamb, or any kind of fish.

INGREDIENTS | MAKES ABOUT 1½ CUPS

1 large mango, peeled, seeded, and diced

1 cup diced fresh pineapple

¼ cup minced red onion

1 teaspoon Tabasco sauce, or to taste

½ teaspoon freshly grated lime zest

Juice of ½ lime

Salt, to taste

Mix together all ingredients in a bowl and cover. Refrigerate for 2 hours. Serve at room temperature.

Crunchy Snack Mix

*To make this recipe dairy-free, just use dairy-free margarine and dairy-free soy cheese.
It's crisp, crunchy, and very satisfying.*

INGREDIENTS | MAKES 8 CUPS

2 cups gluten-free pretzel sticks

2 cups sweet potato chips

1 cup amaranth crackers

1 cup rice chips

2 cups crisp potato sticks

½ cup butter

1 tablespoon gluten-free chili powder

½ teaspoon ground cumin

⅛ teaspoon ground black pepper

½ teaspoon crushed red pepper flakes

½ cup grated Parmesan cheese

1. Preheat oven to 300°F. Slightly crush the pretzel sticks, sweet potato chips, amaranth crackers, and rice chips; combine in a large roasting pan with potato sticks.

2. In small saucepan, melt butter over low heat. Add chili powder, cumin, pepper, and red pepper flakes; remove from heat. Drizzle over ingredients in roasting pan.

3. Bake for 40–50 minutes, stirring twice during baking time, until snack mix is glazed and light golden brown. Sprinkle with cheese, toss to coat, and let cool.

Healthy Snacks

There are so many varieties and brands of specialty snacks available now. Gluten-free crackers, chips, and snack mixes made from rice and potatoes, as well as whole-grain snacks, are commonplace. If you can't find them at your grocery store, ask. Often, the grocer will order items for you. And of course, there's always the Internet.

Grilled Shrimp Skewers

Mustard and lemon juice flavor tender shrimp in this easy recipe. You could use cubes of chicken or turkey instead of the shrimp for a seafood-free recipe.

INGREDIENTS | SERVES 4–6

2 tablespoons olive oil

2 medium onions

2 tablespoons lemon juice

2 tablespoons gluten-free Dijon mustard

½ teaspoon dried thyme leaves

1½ pounds large raw shrimp

½ teaspoon salt

⅛ teaspoon ground black pepper

1. Place olive oil in a medium pan over medium heat. Cut onions into quarters, then cut each quarter in half to make 16 wedges. Cook in oil, turning carefully to keep the wedges together, for 4–5 minutes to soften.

2. Remove pan from heat, then remove onions from pan and set aside. Add lemon juice, mustard, and thyme to olive oil and mix well. Add shrimp and stir to coat.

3. String shrimp and onion wedges on skewers; brush with any remaining mustard mixture and sprinkle with salt and pepper.

4. Cook 6" from broiler or over medium coals, turning once, until shrimp curl and turn pink and onions are slightly charred, about 4–5 minutes. Serve immediately.

Roasted Sweet and Spicy Soybeans

Made in two steps, this wonderful recipe is a great snack for those allergic to nuts.
You can flavor the "nuts" any way you'd like.

INGREDIENTS | SERVES 6

2 cups dried soybeans

6 cups water

1/3 cup honey

1 tablespoon gluten-free curry powder

1 teaspoon fine salt

1. Pick over soybeans, discarding any that are shriveled, along with any extraneous material. Rinse soybeans in cold water, drain, then place in a large bowl. Cover with water and let soak for 12 hours.

2. Preheat oven to 325°F. Drain soybeans and pat dry with paper towels. Place in a single layer on a large baking sheet. Roast for 55–65 minutes, turning with a spatula every 10 minutes, until crisp and light golden brown. Remove from baking sheet; let stand on paper towels for 10 minutes.

3. Return soybeans to baking sheet and drizzle with honey. Toss to coat, then sprinkle with curry powder and salt.

4. Reduce oven temperature to 275°F. Roast the seasoned soybeans another 30–40 minutes, stirring every 8 minutes, until crisp. Let cool, then store in airtight container.

Stuffed Cherry Tomatoes

You can flavor the basic filling any way you'd like: Add jalapeño peppers, chopped toasted nuts, tiny shrimp, cooked ground ham, or pepperoni.

INGREDIENTS | SERVES 12

2 pints cherry tomatoes

1 cup crumbled feta cheese

⅓ cup mayonnaise

1 tablespoon gluten-free prepared horseradish

1 tablespoon lemon juice

¼ cup finely chopped ripe olives, if desired

⅓ cup chopped fresh flat-leaf parsley

¼ cup chopped fresh cilantro

Fresh curly leaf parsley sprigs, for garnish

1. Cut the tops off each cherry tomato; using a small serrated spoon or melon scoop, remove pulp and discard. Put tomatoes upside down on paper towel–lined plates to drain.

2. In a small bowl, combine remaining ingredients and mix well to blend. Spoon or pipe filling into each cherry tomato.

3. To serve, place curly leaf parsley on a serving plate and arrange tomatoes on top. Cover with plastic wrap and chill at least 1 hour before serving.

CHAPTER 14

Smoothies

Berry Banana Smoothie

The delicious combination of bananas, strawberries, and blueberries stars in a smooth and flavorful one-glass wonder. Whether a breakfast treat or an afternoon pick-me-up, this amazing smoothie is sure to be a sensation for the senses.

INGREDIENTS | SERVES 2

2 medium bananas, peeled

1 cup strawberries

1 cup blueberries

1 cup strawberry kefir

1 teaspoon vanilla extract

2 cups ice

1. Combine bananas, berries, kefir, and vanilla extract in a blender with 1 cup ice and blend until thoroughly combined.

2. Add remaining cup of ice gradually while blending until desired consistency is reached.

Packed with Potassium

Although most people indulge in a tasty banana for its creamy, sweet deliciousness, this power fruit does much more than just taste great. It's full of potassium, a necessary mineral that most people don't get enough of. Potassium can even promote cardiovascular health by preventing high blood pressure!

Pumpkin Spice Smoothie

If you're looking for an escape from the usual fruit smoothie, mix things up with this delicious pumpkin pie in a glass! Raw ingredients and aromatic spices make this clean smoothie the most delicious and healthy dessert option around.

INGREDIENTS | SERVES 2

1 cup pumpkin purée

1 cup vanilla almond milk

1 teaspoon ground cloves

1 teaspoon ground ginger

1 teaspoon ground cinnamon

2 cups ice

1. Combine pumpkin, almond milk, and spices in a blender with 1 cup ice and blend until thoroughly combined.

2. Add remaining cup of ice gradually while blending until desired consistency is reached.

Peaches 'n' Cream Smoothie

A creamy combination of delightful peaches, bananas, and almond milk make for a sweet smoothie option. All clean, all healthy, and all absolutely delicious, these ingredients make for a fabulous treat.

INGREDIENTS | SERVES 2

2 cups fresh chopped peaches

1 medium banana, peeled

2 cups vanilla almond milk

2 cups ice

1. Combine peaches, banana, and almond milk in a blender with ½ cup ice and blend until thoroughly combined.

2. Add remaining ice gradually while blending until desired consistency is reached.

Pineapple Delight Smoothie

This smoothie combines the unique flavor of pineapple with delicious coconut milk, making one amazingly light and satisfying treat!

INGREDIENTS | SERVES 2

2 cups fresh pineapple (about 1 large pineapple)

2 cups unsweetened coconut milk

2 cups ice

1. Combine pineapple and coconut milk in a blender with ½ cup ice and blend until thoroughly combined.

2. Add remaining ice gradually while blending until desired consistency is reached.

Pineapple Promotes Health

Pineapples are loaded with valuable vitamins and minerals. Topping the charts for its exceptional doses of manganese, vitamin C, and B vitamins, this is one fruit that's worth its weight in health benefits. Indulging in this sweet fruit provides protection against illness and promotes top brain functioning and quick metabolism—while tasting delicious. What more could you ask for from a beautiful, healthy fruit?

Sour Apple Smoothie

Tart lemons and sweet apples combine in this delicious wake-me-up smoothie that will liven up any sluggish morning or slow-moving day. Whether you prefer to have your smoothies sweet or spicy, this one will surely grab your attention for its unique flavors.

INGREDIENTS | SERVES 2

2 large Granny Smith apples, peeled and cored

1 medium lemon, peeled and seeds removed

1 cup filtered water

1 cup ice

2 tablespoons agave nectar, or to taste

1. Combine apples, lemon, and water in a blender and blend until thoroughly combined with no apple bits remaining.

2. Add ice while blending until desired consistency is achieved.

3. Drizzle in 1 tablespoon agave and blend. Taste and add remaining agave until desired sweetness is achieved.

Mega Melon Smoothie

The cool and lightly sweet refreshment that can only come from fresh melons is bursting out of this smoothie. A great way to add fruit servings to your day, this smoothie is the perfect treat on any hot afternoon.

INGREDIENTS | SERVES 2

½ medium cantaloupe, rind and seeds removed

½ medium honeydew melon, rind and seeds removed

½ cup filtered water

1½ cups ice

1. Combine cantaloupe, honeydew, water, and ½ of the ice in a blender, and blend until thoroughly combined.

2. Add remaining ice while blending until desired consistency is achieved.

Hydrating Melons

Fruit smoothies are a tasty way to hydrate, and including melon in your delicious snack makes them that much more thirst-quenching. Packed with amazing amounts of vitamins and nutrients, this healthy fruit adds tons of hydrating juices to any blended drink!

Beet and Fruit Smoothie

By combining a variety of vibrant colors in your diet, you can ensure you're providing the variety of vitamins and minerals your body requires to run at its optimal level. These ingredients are a treat for your eyes and your body.

INGREDIENTS | SERVES 2

1 cup beet greens

1 medium beet

3 medium carrots, peeled

2 large apples, cored

1 medium banana, peeled

3 cups brewed green tea, divided

1. Combine beet greens, beet, carrots, apples, banana, and 1½ cups tea in a blender and blend until thoroughly combined.

2. Add remaining 1½ cups tea while blending until desired consistency is achieved.

Pomegranate Green Smoothie

Packed with vitamins and minerals that promote health and fight illness, the delicious fruit and vegetables in this smoothie are a tasty way to maintain great health.

INGREDIENTS | SERVES 2

1 cup torn romaine lettuce leaves

2 cups pomegranate pips

1 large orange, peeled

1 medium banana, peeled

1 cup filtered water, divided

1. Combine lettuce, pomegranate, orange, banana, and ½ cup water in a blender and blend until thoroughly combined.

2. Add remaining ½ cup water while blending until desired consistency is achieved.

Ginger and Apple Cleansing Smoothie

Ginger makes a star-studded appearance as a lightly spicy and aromatic addition in this smoothie that is loaded with fiber from the spinach and apples.

INGREDIENTS | SERVES 2

1 cup fresh spinach
3 medium apples, peeled and cored
½" piece fresh gingerroot, peeled
2 cups filtered water, divided

1. Combine spinach, apples, ginger, and 1 cup water in a blender and blend until thoroughly combined.

2. Add remaining water while blending until desired texture is achieved.

The Importance of Fiber

Apples are sometimes referred to as nature's scrub brushes because of the powerful amount of fiber they contain. Found in deep greens, vegetables, and fruit, fiber plays an important role in helping your body rid itself of waste products that may be causing irregularity. The indigestible fibers that pass through the digestive system literally sweep lingering waste with them as they leave the body.

Savory Green Smoothie

This colorful combination of vegetables makes a visually and palate-pleasing creation. The ingredients provide a wealth of vitamins and minerals that will optimize digestive health and comfort.

INGREDIENTS | SERVES 2

1 cup spinach

1 cup asparagus spears

½ lemon, peeled

1 medium tomato

1–2 cloves garlic, depending upon size

2 cups filtered water, divided

1. Combine spinach, asparagus, lemon, tomato, garlic, and 1 cup water in a blender and blend until thoroughly combined.

2. Add remaining 1 cup of water while blending until desired texture is achieved.

Eat the Rainbow for Optimal Health

It may be difficult to figure out which food group is best for your body and promoting its ideal functioning. The answer is . . . all of them! The easiest route to achieving optimum health is to eat the rainbow: Eat a variety of different foods with vibrant colors. By consuming a variety of fruit and vegetables with color, you can ensure your body is receiving abundant vitamins and nutrients. With variety comes the added benefit of never becoming tired of the same old fruit or veggie.

Amazing Avocado Smoothie

If you're looking to add the good fats that can be found in nuts, seeds, and certain fruit to your diet, avocados should definitely be in your kitchen. The creamy texture of avocados makes a perfect addition to salads, soups, and smoothies.

INGREDIENTS | SERVES 2

1 cup spinach

2 medium avocados, peeled and seeds removed

1 large lime, peeled

1 cup filtered water, divided

1 cup plain vegan Greek-style yogurt, divided

1. Combine spinach, avocados, lime, ½ cup water, and ½ cup yogurt in a blender and blend until thoroughly combined.

2. Add remaining ½ cup water and ½ cup yogurt while blending until desired texture is achieved.

Avocados and Oral Cancer

Although avocados have been found to fight the cancer-causing free radicals of colon, breast, and prostate cancers, the most notable protective benefit avocados create in the human body is the protection against oral cancer. With a 50 percent mortality rate most commonly due to late detection, oral cancer is a preventable cancer that can be helped with the addition of just 2 ounces of avocado per day to your diet.

Cocoa Banana Smoothie

*Bursting with flavor, this smoothie provides more nutrition than you would think.
Vitamins, minerals, and antioxidants beam from each ingredient!*

INGREDIENTS | SERVES 2

1 cup torn romaine lettuce leaves
2 medium bananas, peeled
1 tablespoon raw cocoa powder
Pulp of ½ vanilla bean
2 cups almond milk, divided

1. Combine romaine, bananas, cocoa powder, vanilla bean pulp, and 1 cup almond milk in a blender and blend until thoroughly combined.

2. Add remaining 1 cup almond milk while blending until desired texture is achieved.

Strawberry Dandelion Smoothie

If you love strawberries, you'll be happy to enjoy it while also fulfilling your daily requirement for an entire serving of greens. Agave nectar comes into this smoothie to sweeten the flavor, but only if desired.

INGREDIENTS | SERVES 2

½ cup dandelion greens

2 pints strawberries

1 cup vanilla soymilk, divided

1 tablespoon agave nectar, or to taste (optional)

Strawberries for Sight

Rich in the antioxidants that give them their vibrant red color, this sweet berry is also rich in vitamins A, C, D, and E; B vitamins; folate; and phytochemicals that join forces to help you maintain healthy eyes and strong vision. Strawberries also may help delay the onset of macular degeneration.

1. Add dandelion greens, strawberries, and ½ cup soymilk in a blender and blend until combined.

2. Slowly add remaining ½ cup soymilk while blending until desired consistency is achieved.

3. Stop blending periodically to check for desired sweetness, and if using, drizzle in agave nectar until desired sweetness is achieved.

Pear and Ginger Smoothie

This refreshing smoothie makes a great snack when your body and mind need a lift. The sweet pears, spicy ginger, and rich cabbage and celery combine with the cooling cucumber for an overall refreshing blend.

INGREDIENTS | SERVES 2

1 cup green cabbage

3 medium pears, cored

1 medium cucumber, peeled

1 medium stalk celery

½" piece fresh gingerroot, peeled

1 cup kefir, divided

1. Combine cabbage, pears, cucumber, celery, ginger, and ½ cup kefir in a blender and blend until thoroughly combined.

2. Add remaining ½ cup kefir while blending until desired consistency is achieved.

Blackberry Lemon Smoothie

Delicious blackberries are made even more tasty with the addition of lemon and ginger in this recipe. This smoothie packs a healthy dose of much-needed vitamins and minerals, and is rich and satisfying with the addition of protein-packed yogurt.

INGREDIENTS | SERVES 2

1 cup watercress
2 pints blackberries
1 medium banana, peeled
½ lemon, peeled
½" piece fresh gingerroot, peeled
1 cup plain Greek-style yogurt, divided

1. Combine watercress, blackberries, banana, lemon, ginger, and ½ cup yogurt in a blender and blend until thoroughly combined.

2. Add remaining ½ cup yogurt while blending until desired consistency is achieved.

Blackberries Promote Respiratory Relief

Rich blackberries are a tasty treat, and they are also packed with a variety of vitamins and minerals that can aid in overall health. Specifically, the magnesium content in blackberries is what makes it a crusader in promoting respiratory ease. Best known for its ability to relax the muscles and thin mucus most commonly associated with breathing difficulties, blackberries are an important addition to those in need of breathing assistance.

CHAPTER 15

Juices

Spicy Melon Juice

Drink a juice made with fresh ginger as soon as you start to feel the symptoms of a migraine.

INGREDIENTS | SERVES 1

½ cantaloupe, peeled
¼" piece fresh gingerroot
½ lemon, peeled

Juice cantaloupe, gingerroot, and lemon. Stir before serving.

Blackberry Banana Juice

The banana in this drink provides the potassium you need when exercising. Potassium is essential for helping muscles contract properly during exercise and reduce cramping.

INGREDIENTS | SERVES 1

2 pints blackberries

½ lemon, peeled

1 medium banana

Juice blackberries and lemon. Add banana and blend until smooth.

Cabbage Juice

Mixing apples and carrots with cabbage sweetens this juice.
Cabbage is high in vitamins C and K, fiber, and detoxifying sulfur compounds.

INGREDIENTS | SERVES 1

1 cup chopped green cabbage
2 medium carrots, peeled
2 large apples, cored

Juice cabbage, carrots, and apples. Stir before serving.

The Canker Sore Connection

Studies show people with celiac disease and frequent yeast infections are more prone to canker sores than others. If you suspect you suffer from either condition, see your physician. A positive diagnosis may lead you to change your diet, which will make you feel like an entirely new person.

Tropical Cucumber Juice

This drink provides skin benefits. Cucumber contains silica, a trace mineral that helps provide strength to the connective tissues of the skin. Cucumbers help with swelling of the eyes and water retention. They are high in vitamins A and C and folic acid.

INGREDIENTS | SERVES 1

1 cup pineapple, peeled and cut into chunks

1 medium mango, pitted

1 large cucumber, peeled

½ large lemon, rind intact

Juice pineapple first, then mango and cucumber. Cut lemon into thin slices and juice it last. Stir well before serving.

Apple Lemonade

Apples are available year round, but are best September through November. Select firm apples with good color. Skins should be smooth and have no blemishes.

INGREDIENTS | SERVES 1

2 red Gala apples, cored
2 Granny Smith apples, cored
¼ large lemon, rind intact

Juice apples first. Cut lemon into thin slices and then juice. Stir before serving.

Peach Strawberry Juice

Peaches bruise easily. Look for intensely fragrant fruit that is soft, and avoid peaches that have green on them.

INGREDIENTS | SERVES 1

1 large peach, pitted

7 large strawberries, hulls intact

Juice peach and then strawberries. Stir before serving.

White Grape and Lime Juice

Look for fresh green grapes that have a pale color for this cool summer drink.

INGREDIENTS | SERVES 1

1½ cups green seedless grapes
2 medium limes, peeled

Juice grapes and limes. Stir before serving.

Cranberry Apple Juice

Cranberries are high in vitamin C. They're only in season for a few months, but fresh berries purchased in November and December can be frozen and used throughout the year.

INGREDIENTS | SERVES 1

1¼ cups cranberries
2 medium red apples, cored

Juice cranberries and apples. Stir before serving.

Pear Pineapple Juice

Pears are a great source of fiber and pectin, both of which are highly beneficial for gut health. Pineapple has long been known for its ability to help with digestion.

INGREDIENTS | SERVES 1

½ pineapple, skin and core removed
2 medium Bartlett pears, cored
1 large lemon, peeled

Juice pineapple, pear, and lemon. Stir before serving.

Seven-Vegetable Juice

This combination of vegetables is so much fresher than anything you can purchase in a canned or bottled juice. Try swapping in more of your favorite vegetables to boost flavor and nutrition.

INGREDIENTS | SERVES 1

2 Roma tomatoes
1 medium stalk celery, leaves intact
1 fistful fresh flat-leaf parsley
2 medium carrots, peeled
1 green onion
1 cup cauliflower florets
2 cloves garlic

Blanch tomatoes by placing in boiling water for 30 seconds and then transferring to an ice bath. Juice ingredients in the order listed. Stir before serving.

The Benefits of Lycopene

Lycopene is a powerful antioxidant found in tomatoes. It has been shown to reduce the risk of prostate, ovarian, and cervical cancer. To reap the benefits of lycopene, the tomatoes must be eaten cooked rather than raw.

Carrot Cauliflower Juice

*This tasty juice provides you with iron and vitamins A and C.
Try using orange cauliflower in this juice for a brighter color.*

INGREDIENTS | SERVES 1

1 cup cauliflower florets
3 medium carrots, peeled
1 medium stalk celery

Juice cauliflower, carrots, and celery. Stir before serving.

Cauliflower or Cabbage?

Mark Twain said, "Cauliflower is nothing but cabbage with a college education." It is part of the cabbage family and comes from the Latin word *caulis* for "stalk" and *floris* for "flower." Cauliflower comes in white, orange, green, and purple varieties. The green leaves at the base of the cauliflower are edible. They have a stronger flavor than the curd.

Broccoli Apple Carrot Juice

Broccoli is now considered one of the top cancer prevention foods by the American Cancer Society—and this juice is packed with nutrients and fresh broccoli flavor.

INGREDIENTS | SERVES 1

4 large broccoli stalks
¼ cup fresh flat-leaf parsley
2 medium McIntosh apples, cored
¼ large lemon

Juice broccoli, parsley, and apples. Juice lemon. Stir before serving.

Spicy Tomato Juice

Research shows that drinking a glass of tomato juice as your first course can cause you to eat up to 135 fewer calories in the rest of your meal.

INGREDIENTS | SERVES 1

6 Roma tomatoes

¼ red onion

½ jalapeño pepper

1 clove garlic

1 medium stalk celery

Juice ingredients in order listed. Stir before serving.

Tomato Juice

Tomato juice was served for the first time in 1917 at a spa in Indiana. A French chef ran out of oranges for orange juice, so he squeezed tomatoes instead. It was a huge success and tomato juice became a popular morning drink.

Root Vegetable Juice

Turnips are packed with cancer-fighting compounds, are rich in the minerals calcium and iron, and have two times the vitamin C of orange juice.

INGREDIENTS | SERVES 1

2 medium carrots, peeled

1 cup spinach

1 medium turnip

1 medium stalk celery

2 sprigs fresh flat-leaf parsley

Juice carrots, spinach, turnip, and celery. Stir and garnish with parsley sprigs.

Healthy Carrots

Carrots have been known for more than 2,000 years for their good health properties and high vitamin A content. They appear in many juice recipes because they are so healthy. They juice well, and complement the flavors of other fruit and vegetables quite nicely.

Pepper Apple Juice

Bell peppers were named for their shape. Sweet peppers come in many different colors, including yellow, red, orange, green, and even purple. They have a mild and sweet flavor, and are excellent sources of vitamins C and A.

INGREDIENTS | SERVES 1

2 medium red apples, cored
1 medium bell pepper

Juice apples and pepper. Stir before serving.

CHAPTER 16

Vegetarian

Scrambled Eggs Masala

These Indian-style eggs have a fragrant allure. Serve them with Curried Cauliflower (see recipe in Chapter 17) and sliced mango for a special brunch.

INGREDIENTS | SERVES 2

2 tablespoons butter

¼ cup chopped onion

¼ teaspoon cumin seed, toasted in a dry pan and crushed (or very fresh ground cumin, toasted in a dry pan)

¼ cup diced tomato

4 large eggs, beaten

Salt and ground white pepper, to taste

4 teaspoons chopped fresh mint leaves

1. Melt butter in a medium nonstick skillet over medium heat.

2. Add onions and cook for 5–8 minutes, until soft. Add cumin and tomatoes and cook 1 minute more.

3. Stir in eggs, salt, and pepper. Using a wooden spoon, constantly stir the eggs until they form soft, creamy curds.

4. Transfer to plates and serve immediately. Garnish with mint.

Huevos Rancheros

Rich and delicious, this Mexican ranch breakfast will fuel your whole morning.
While this recipe calls for scrambled eggs, it works equally well with any style of eggs.

INGREDIENTS | SERVES 4

1 (15-ounce) can Mexican-style black beans in sauce

2 cups salsa

8 large eggs

½ cup half-and-half

½ teaspoon salt

2 tablespoons unsalted butter

8 (6") soft corn tortillas

1 cup shredded Monterey jack or mild Cheddar cheese

½ cup sour cream

Chopped fresh cilantro, to taste

Softening Store-Bought Tortillas

Right from the package, some corn tortillas may be cardboardy and mealy. They should be exposed to either dry or moist heat for a minute before serving. This is done either by steaming them for 1 minute, one at a time, in a standard steamer basket, or by placing them directly onto the burner of a gas stove, allowing the flames to lightly brown the tortillas on both sides. You'll notice a definite "puff" in most tortillas when properly softened. Another alternative is to toast them briefly in a toaster oven.

1. Heat beans and salsa in separate small saucepans over low heat.

2. In a large bowl, whisk together eggs, half-and-half, and salt.

3. Melt butter in a large nonstick skillet over low heat. Pour egg mixture into the skillet. Using a wooden spoon, constantly stir until the eggs form soft, small, creamy curds.

4. Soften tortillas either by steaming or flash cooking over an open gas burner (see sidebar instructions).

5. Place 2 tortillas onto each plate. Divide the hot black beans evenly onto the tortillas. Spoon the eggs onto the beans, then sauce with a ladleful of salsa.

6. Garnish with cheese, sour cream, and cilantro. Serve immediately.

Smoky Black-Eyed Pea Soup with Butternut Squash and Mustard Greens

Black-eyed peas offer some of the delicious earthiness of green peas, but also a savory touch. Use any dark leafy greens you'd like, fresh or frozen, in place of the mustard greens.

INGREDIENTS | SERVES 10–12

1 tablespoon olive oil

1 medium onion, chopped

2 medium stalks celery, chopped

1 medium carrot, peeled and chopped

2 teaspoons salt

1 teaspoon dried thyme

2 teaspoons dried oregano

1 teaspoon ground cumin

1 dried chipotle chili, halved

2 dried bay leaves

1 pound dried black-eyed peas or navy beans, washed and picked through for stones

2 quarts Vegetable Stock (see recipe in Chapter 11) or water

½ large butternut squash, peeled and diced into 1" cubes

1 (10-ounce) package frozen mustard greens, chopped

1 (28-ounce) can diced tomatoes

Fresh chopped cilantro, for garnish

1. In a large, heavy-bottomed Dutch oven heat oil over medium heat for 1 minute. Add onion, celery, carrot, and salt and cook for about 5 minutes, until onion is translucent.

2. Add thyme, oregano, cumin, chipotle chili, and bay leaves and cook for 2 minutes more.

3. Add black-eyed peas and vegetable stock. Bring to a boil, then reduce to a simmer; cook for 2 hours, or until beans are very tender, adding more stock or water if necessary.

4. Add squash and cook 20 minutes more. Stir in chopped mustard greens and diced tomatoes. Cook 10 minutes more, until the squash and greens are tender.

5. Adjust seasoning with salt and pepper, and consistency with additional vegetable stock or water as desired. The soup should be brothy.

6. Remove bay leaves. Serve garnished with a sprinkling of chopped cilantro.

Vegan Chili

This hearty warm-up is especially delicious served over warm brown rice.

INGREDIENTS | SERVES 8

¼ cup olive oil

2 cups chopped yellow onion

1 cup peeled and chopped carrot

2 cups chopped assorted bell peppers

2 teaspoons salt

1 tablespoon chopped garlic

2 jalapeño peppers, seeded and chopped

1 tablespoon ground ancho chili pepper or ½ teaspoon crushed red pepper flakes

1 chipotle in adobo, chopped

1 tablespoon cumin seed, toasted in a dry pan and ground, or 4 teaspoons ground cumin, toasted briefly in a dry pan

1 (28-ounce) can plum tomatoes, roughly chopped, juice included

3 (15-ounce) cans beans: 1 each red kidney, cannellini, and black beans, rinsed and drained

1 cup tomato juice

Finely chopped red onion, for garnish

Chopped fresh cilantro, for garnish

1. Heat oil in a large Dutch oven or heavy-bottomed soup pot. Add onion, carrot, bell peppers, and salt and cook for 15 minutes over medium heat, until the onions are soft.

2. Add garlic, jalapeños, ancho, chipotle, and cumin and cook 5 minutes more.

3. Stir in tomatoes, beans, and tomato juice. Simmer for 45 minutes.

4. Serve garnished with red onions and cilantro.

A Mexican Pantry

Key items for your Mexican-inspired pantry include pickled jalapeño peppers, chipotle (smoked chilies) in adobo (tomato-based sauce), nopales (pronounced "noh-*pah*-lays"; slices of delicious cactus perfect in salads, stews, and wraps), and Mexican chocolate disks (the best hot chocolate you'll ever taste—it's made with cinnamon bark and ground almonds). If your local specialty store is lacking, find them online!

Egyptian Lentils and Rice

*Amino acids in the lentils and rice combine to form complete proteins,
making this warming, comforting dish nutritionally powerful.*

INGREDIENTS | SERVES 8

1 tablespoon olive oil

¼ teaspoon cumin seed

1 medium onion, roughly chopped

1 cup brown rice

½ cup brown or green lentils

2 teaspoons lemon juice

½ teaspoon lemon zest

1 teaspoon salt

3 cups Vegetable Stock (see recipe in Chapter 11) or water

1. Heat oil and cumin seed in a medium saucepan over medium heat until cumin is fragrant, about 30 seconds. Add onion and cook until translucent, about 5 minutes.

2. Stir in rice and lentils, mixing with a wooden spoon until well coated. Add lemon juice, zest, salt, and stock. Cover tightly and simmer until all water is absorbed, about 20 minutes.

3. Remove from heat and let stand for 5 minutes before fluffing with a fork and serving.

4. Optional: This dish is delicious served with a dab of Egyptian chili sauce (harissa) or other chili paste.

Rinsing Rice

To make perfect rice, start by washing the grains thoroughly under running water. Try pouring as much rice as you plan to use into the pot you plan to cook it in, and run cold water over the rice, agitating it with your hand until the water is no longer cloudy, but runs clear. This washes off excess starch on the outside of the grains, eliminates any pesticides that may have been used wherever the rice was warehoused (especially important with Indian basmati rice), and rinses off any other unwanted residue.

Spinach-Stuffed Vegetables

The little child in all of us loves stuffed things—maybe it's just the sneaky feeling that we're getting two things instead of just one. But the best reason to treasure this colorful cornucopia is that it's easy to make.

INGREDIENTS | SERVES 4

1 tablespoon olive oil

1 tablespoon coriander seed

3 medium shallots, roughly chopped

¼ teaspoon crushed red pepper flakes (optional)

2 pounds spinach, stemmed

½ teaspoon salt

¼ cup crumbled feta cheese

4 plum tomatoes, tops cut off, insides scooped out

1 medium zucchini, cut into 4 (2") cylinders

1 medium yellow squash, cut into 4 (2") cylinders

4 large cremini mushrooms, stems removed

Salt and ground white pepper, to taste

Lemon wedges, for garnish

1. Heat olive oil and coriander in a small pan until very hot but not smoking; the coriander should become fragrant, but not brown. Strain the oil into a large skillet or Dutch oven; discard seeds.

2. Place the skillet or Dutch oven over medium heat. Add shallots and crushed pepper (if using) and cook for 1 minute; they should sizzle but not brown.

3. Add spinach all at once; season with salt and cook, stirring, just until spinach is wilted. Transfer to a colander to cool.

4. Chop the spinach roughly on a cutting board and return to the pan. Add feta cheese.

5. Trim the bottoms of the tomatoes just enough to help them stand straight. Using a small spoon or melon baller, scoop enough of the seeded center from the zucchini and yellow squash to form a teaspoon-sized pocket. Season the zucchini, squash, and mushrooms liberally with salt and white pepper.

6. Spoon the spinach mixture into the vegetables, mounding slightly on top. Any extra spinach may be used to line the plates when serving.

7. Arrange the vegetables in a steamer basket. Steam over rapidly boiling water just until the zucchini become tender, about 6 minutes. Serve hot or at room temperature, along with remaining spinach filling and lemon wedges.

Pickled Mushrooms

As a snack or as part of a dinner buffet, pickled mushrooms bring an attractive piquancy to the table. They keep refrigerated for weeks.

INGREDIENTS | SERVES 8

1½ pounds small white mushrooms, halved

3 medium carrots, peeled and cut into julienne

1 tablespoon olive oil

½ cup canned pimientos, cut into 1" × ½" strips

½ teaspoon dried oregano

½ teaspoon garlic powder

¼ cup apple cider vinegar

½ teaspoon salt

¼ teaspoon ground black pepper

1. Boil mushrooms and carrots in separate pots until fork-tender and then drain.

2. Heat oil in a medium skillet and add carrots. Cook for 3 minutes. Add mushrooms and cook for 3 minutes more, then add pimiento, oregano, garlic powder, cider vinegar, salt, and pepper.

3. Cook until everything is heated through. Refrigerate for 24 hours before serving.

What Are Truffles?

Truffles are so special, only pigs and dogs can find them! Truffles are fragrant underground fungi related to mushrooms. Their musky aroma is heavenly to some. Extremely expensive due to their rarity and inability to be cultivated, they are sold fresh, dried, or canned, usually imported from France or Italy. The Italian white truffle from Alba is the most highly prized, and is worth, literally, more than its weight in gold. Like black truffles from France, the Alba truffle is usually shaved paper-thin over simple foods like pasta, polenta, or eggs, the better to appreciate its rare character.

Creamed Carrots

There should be a dynamic array of colors, textures, and flavors in any meal you prepare. With their appealing color and gentle bite, these carrots supply both elements. Also, since the vitamin A in carrots is lipid soluble, this ingredient combination aids in the release of this important nutrient.

INGREDIENTS | SERVES 4

1 pound carrots
½ cup water
2 tablespoons unsalted butter
1½ teaspoons granulated sugar
½ teaspoon salt
½ cup light cream
Pinch grated nutmeg
Ground white pepper, to taste (optional)

1. Peel carrots, quarter lengthwise, and cut into 2" sticks.

2. Combine carrots, water, butter, sugar, and salt in a large skillet. Simmer over medium heat until most of the water has evaporated and carrots are tender.

3. Add cream. Simmer until it lightly coats the carrots and has a saucy consistency.

4. Season carrots with nutmeg and white pepper, if desired.

Spinach and Tomato Sauté

The subtle addition of coriander brings this dish an understated elegance, perfect for a dinner main course. Always wash spinach twice, submerging it in fresh water each time and agitating it well by hand. Because it grows low to the ground, spinach usually hides plenty of soil in its crevices.

INGREDIENTS | SERVES 4

3 teaspoons butter, divided

6 plum tomatoes, roughly chopped

1 teaspoon ground coriander

2 large bunches spinach

½ teaspoon salt

Freshly ground black pepper, to taste

1. In a large skillet or heavy-bottomed Dutch oven, melt 2 teaspoons butter over medium-high heat. Add tomatoes and coriander; cook until softened, about 5 minutes.

2. Add spinach in handfuls, allowing each handful to wilt before adding the next. Season well with salt and pepper.

3. Finish by adding the remaining butter to the pan and allowing it to melt, mixing with spinach.

Nonreactive Pots: Welcome to the Steel and Glass Generation

Aluminum and copper, commonly used materials in pots and pans, react with (and alter the flavor and color of) acidic foods. Always use pans with a stainless steel or glass cooking surface to avoid sour tomato sauce, discolored green beans, and "off"-tasting soups. For the lightweight and even heat of aluminum and copper, combined with the nonreactive property of steel, buy aluminum or copper alloy pots clad to a steel "jacket" (inner lining).

Garlicky Broccoli Raab

The key to the toasty flavor of this dish is to brown the garlic to a golden color before adding the blanched raab. Their moisture stops the garlic from cooking, preserving its browned, but not burned flavor.

INGREDIENTS | SERVES 4

1 pound broccoli raab, bottoms trimmed

2 tablespoons good-quality olive oil

2 tablespoons finely chopped garlic

Pinch crushed red pepper flakes (optional)

Salt and freshly ground black pepper, to taste

Lemon wedges, for garnish

Spicy Variations

In place of or in addition to pepper flakes, substitute toasted cumin seed, fennel seed, anise, or chopped fresh ginger for different character.

1. Blanch raab in rapidly boiling salted water, then shock in ice water and drain.

2. Heat olive oil in a large, heavy-bottomed skillet over medium heat for 1 minute. Add garlic and red pepper flakes, if using, and cook, stirring with a wooden spoon until garlic is golden, about 5 minutes.

3. Add all the raab at once; toss to coat. Heat through and season with salt and pepper (making sure to taste as you season, remembering that the raab was blanched in salted water).

4. Serve with lemon wedges on the side.

Swiss Chard Ravioli

These ravioli are excellent with a simple fresh tomato sauce and freshly grated Parmesan cheese.

INGREDIENTS | SERVES 8

2 tablespoons olive oil

1 medium onion, finely chopped

1 tablespoon chopped garlic (2–3 cloves)

Pinch crushed red pepper flakes (optional)

1 large bunch (about 1½ pounds) red or green Swiss chard, stems removed

12 ounces (1½ cups) ricotta cheese

½ cup grated Parmigiano-Reggiano or Asiago cheese (use top quality)

1 tablespoon gluten-free bread crumbs

2 beaten eggs, divided

Salt and freshly ground black pepper, to taste

4 (9" × 14") sheets gluten-free pasta dough

Mushroom Sauce for Your Swiss Chard Ravioli

Another delicious way to serve this ravioli dish is with exotic mushrooms in brown butter: Cook 1 stick of butter in a large skillet over medium heat until lightly browned, then add 2 cups sliced shiitake mushrooms and ½ teaspoon of salt, and cook for 2 minutes. Squeeze in juice of ½ lemon, and spoon over the hot ravioli immediately before serving. Sprinkle with chopped fresh Italian flat-leaf parsley.

1. Heat oil in a large skillet over medium-high heat. Add onion, garlic, and red pepper, if using, and cook for 5 minutes until onion is translucent. Add chard; cook until just wilted. Transfer to a colander to cool and drain.

2. Once chard has cooled, squeeze out excess moisture with your hands. Transfer to a cutting board and give it a rough chopping.

3. In a large mixing bowl, combine chopped chard, ricotta, Parmigiano-Reggiano, bread crumbs, and half the eggs. Season to taste with salt and black pepper (season it highly, as you'll only use a little in each ravioli).

4. Place 12 evenly spaced, tablespoon-sized dabs of filling onto each of 2 pasta sheets. Use a pastry brush to paint in between the filling portions with the remaining egg.

5. Loosely cover these pasta sheets with the remaining 2 sheets. Press down with your hands to squeeze out any air pockets, and press firmly to seal in the filling.

6. Using a knife, or fluted pastry cutter, cut between the ravioli, separating them, and pinch the edges extra tight between your fingers. Allow them to dry for 15–30 minutes before cooking in rapidly boiling salted water.

Fennel with Lemon and Parmesan

This simple but delicious snack typifies the essence of Italian cuisine:
Use the best ingredients without overcomplicating them.

INGREDIENTS | SERVES 4

2 large bulbs fresh fennel

½ large lemon

1 wedge (at least 4" long) Parmigiano-Reggiano cheese or Asiago cheese

1 tablespoon high-quality extra-virgin olive oil

Pinch salt

Even-Seasoning Secret

To avoid salty patches in some parts of your food and bland, unseasoned patches on other parts, take a cue from pro chefs: Season from a great height. Most chefs pinch salt between their thumb and forefinger and sprinkle it down onto food from more than a foot above the item being seasoned. It tends to shower broadly over the food this way, covering evenly.

1. Trim stems and hairlike fronds from fennel tops. Break bulbs apart, layer by layer, using your hands to make long, bite-sized pieces. Discard the core. Arrange the pieces pyramid-shape onto a small, attractive serving plate.

2. Squeeze lemon over the fennel. Using a peeler, shave curls of cheese over the top, allowing them to fall where they may; make about 10 curls.

3. Drizzle olive oil over the plate, and sprinkle with salt. Serve at room temperature.

Smooth Cauliflower Soup with Coriander

This no-cream "cream soup" is equally delicious hot or chilled.

INGREDIENTS | SERVES 4–6

2 tablespoons unsalted butter or olive oil

1 medium onion, chopped

2 tablespoons white wine or dry sherry

1 medium head (about 2 pounds) cauliflower, cut into bite-sized pieces

2 cups Vegetable Stock (see recipe in Chapter 11)

1 teaspoon salt

Ground white pepper, to taste

1 teaspoon ground coriander

¾ cup cold whole milk, divided

Chopped fresh chives or flat-leaf parsley, for garnish

1. In a large saucepan or soup pot, melt butter over medium-high heat. Add onion and cook until translucent but not brown, about 5 minutes.

2. Add wine and cauliflower and cook for 1 minute to steam out the alcohol. Add stock, salt, pepper, and coriander and bring to a rolling boil.

3. Simmer until cauliflower is very tender, about 15 minutes.

4. Transfer to a blender. Add half the milk and purée until very smooth, scraping down the sides of the blender vase with a rubber spatula. Be careful during this step, since hot liquids will splash out of the blender if it is not started gradually (you may wish to purée in 2 batches for safety).

5. Transfer soup back to saucepan, and thin with additional milk if necessary. Adjust seasoning to taste and garnish with chopped chives or parsley just before serving.

Spiced Pecans

These irresistible, fragrant pecans make a beautiful holiday gift wrapped up in decorative tins. Or, try serving at Thanksgiving as an appetizer or as a topping to green salad.

INGREDIENTS | MAKES 3 CUPS

2 tablespoons unsalted butter

1 pound whole, shelled pecans

2 tablespoons light gluten-free soy sauce

1 tablespoon hoisin sauce

A few drops of hot pepper sauce

1. Heat oven to 325°F. Melt butter in a large skillet. Add nuts and cook, tossing occasionally, until nuts are well coated.

2. Add soy sauce, hoisin sauce, and hot pepper sauce and cook 1 minute more. Stir to coat thoroughly.

3. Spread nuts into a single layer on a baking sheet. Bake until all liquid is absorbed and nuts begin to brown. Remove from oven. Cool before serving.

Honey-Orange Beets

If you are able to find fresh beets with the greens still attached, wash them thoroughly, dress them with lemon and olive oil, and use them as a bed for this dish, creating a warm-salad main course.

INGREDIENTS | SERVES 4

6 medium beets

1 teaspoon grated orange zest

2 tablespoons orange juice

2 teaspoons butter

1 teaspoon honey

¼ teaspoon ground ginger

Salt and freshly ground black pepper, to taste

1. Boil beets in enough water to cover for 40 minutes, or until tender. Drain beets and let cool slightly. Slip off skins and slice.

2. In a medium saucepan, heat orange zest, orange juice, butter, honey, and ginger over low heat until the butter melts. Add beets and toss to coat. Season with salt and pepper.

Cooking Beets—Preserving Nutrition

The flavorful, nutrient-rich juices in beets are water soluble. To lock in the sweetness, color, and food value of these wonderful vegetables, consider cooking them in their skins. When boiling them, put a few drops of red wine vinegar in the water, which also helps seal in beet juices. Beets can also be baked whole, like potatoes, then peeled and sliced.

CHAPTER 17

Slow Cooker

Creamy Chickpea Soup

Beans can be puréed to make a creamy soup without the cream.

INGREDIENTS | SERVES 6

1 small onion, diced

2 cloves garlic, minced

2 (15-ounce) cans chickpeas, drained and rinsed

5 cups Vegetable Stock (see recipe in Chapter 11)

1 teaspoon salt

½ teaspoon ground cumin

Juice of ½ medium lemon

1 tablespoon olive oil

¼ cup chopped fresh flat-leaf parsley

1. In a 4-quart slow cooker, add all ingredients except lemon juice, olive oil, and parsley. Cover, and cook over low heat for 4 hours.

2. Allow to cool slightly, then process the soup in a blender—carefully, in batches—or by using an immersion blender.

3. Return the soup to the slow cooker; add lemon juice, olive oil, and parsley, and heat on low for an additional 30 minutes.

Étouffée

This spicy, aromatic Cajun and Creole dish is typically served with shellfish, like crawfish or shrimp, over rice.

INGREDIENTS | SERVES 6

½ cup butter

1 medium onion, diced

3 medium stalks celery, chopped

1 medium carrot, peeled and diced

3 cloves garlic, minced

1 medium green bell pepper, chopped

¼ cup gluten-free flour

1 cup water

2 teaspoons Cajun seasoning

Juice of 1 large lemon

½ teaspoon salt

¼ teaspoon ground black pepper

1 pound crawfish or medium shrimp, peeled and deveined

4 cups cooked brown rice

½ cup chopped fresh flat-leaf parsley

1. In a medium sauté pan, heat butter over medium heat. Sauté onion, celery, carrot, garlic, and green bell pepper until soft, about 5–7 minutes. Stir in flour to make a roux, whisking to prevent clumps.

2. Add the vegetable mixture to a 4-quart slow cooker. Whisk in water, Cajun seasoning, lemon juice, salt, and pepper. Cover and cook on low heat for 4–5 hours.

3. The last 30 minutes of cooking, add the crawfish or shrimp. (Seafood will be ready to serve when it is opaque, pink, and tender.)

4. Serve over brown rice and garnish with parsley.

Cajun Seasoning

To make your own Cajun seasoning, use a blend of equal parts cayenne pepper, black pepper, paprika, garlic powder, onion powder, salt, and thyme.

Fajita Chili

Re-create the flavor of sizzling restaurant fajitas in your own home!

INGREDIENTS | SERVES 6

1 medium red onion, diced

1 medium jalapeño, seeded and minced

3 cloves garlic, minced

1 (15-ounce) can black beans, drained and rinsed

1 (15-ounce) can diced tomatoes, drained and rinsed

1 pound cooked chicken breasts, cut into bite-sized pieces

2 cups Chicken Broth (see recipe in Chapter 11)

2 teaspoons chili powder

1 teaspoon granulated sugar

1 teaspoon paprika

¼ teaspoon garlic powder

¼ teaspoon ground cayenne pepper

¼ teaspoon ground cumin

1 teaspoon salt

¼ teaspoon ground black pepper

1. In a 4-quart slow cooker, combine all ingredients.

2. Cover and cook on low heat for 5 hours.

Simplify This Recipe

One way to simplify this recipe is to use a packet of fajita seasoning (sold in the international aisle in many stores) in place of the chili powder, sugar, paprika, garlic powder, cayenne pepper, cumin, salt, and black pepper. Be wary of sodium levels, however; some prepackaged seasoning mixes contain high levels of salt.

Tomato Basil Soup

*Fresh basil adds a different flavor than dried basil to dishes,
and the fresh variety is more complementary to this soup.*

INGREDIENTS | SERVES 5

2 tablespoons butter

½ medium onion, diced

2 cloves garlic, minced

1 (28-ounce) can whole peeled tomatoes

½ cup Vegetable Stock (see recipe in Chapter 11)

1 dried bay leaf

1 teaspoon salt

1 teaspoon ground black pepper

½ cup unsweetened soymilk

¼ cup sliced fresh basil

1. In a large sauté pan over medium heat, melt butter; sauté onion and garlic for 3–4 minutes.

2. In a 4-quart slow cooker, add onion and garlic, tomatoes, stock, bay leaf, salt, and pepper. Cover and cook on low heat 4 hours.

3. Allow to cool slightly, then remove the bay leaf. Process the soup in a blender—carefully, in batches— or using an immersion blender.

4. Return the soup to the slow cooker; add soymilk and chopped basil, and heat on low for an additional 30 minutes.

Pork Steaks in Apple and Prune Sauce

Serve this dish over tender brown rice and alongside Garlicky Broccoli Raab (see recipe in Chapter 16).

INGREDIENTS | SERVES 6

12 pitted prunes

3 pounds boneless pork steaks, trimmed of fat

2 Granny Smith apples, peeled, cored, and sliced

¾ cup dry white wine or apple juice

¾ cup heavy cream

Salt and freshly ground black pepper, to taste

1 tablespoon red currant jelly

1 tablespoon butter, divided (optional)

1. Add prunes, pork steaks, apple slices, wine or apple juice, and cream to a 4-quart or larger slow cooker. Add salt and pepper to taste. Cover and cook on low for 6 hours.

2. Now you have a choice: You can either remove the meat and fruit to a serving platter and keep warm, or you can just remove the meat, skim the fat from the liquid in the slow cooker, and use an immersion blender to blend the fruit into the creamy broth.

3. Cook uncovered on high for 30 minutes or until the pan juices begin to bubble around the edges. Reduce the setting to low or simmer, and cook for 15 more minutes or until the mixture is reduced by half and thickened.

4. Whisk in red currant jelly. Taste for seasoning and add more salt and pepper if needed. Whisk in butter 1 teaspoon at a time if you want a richer, glossier sauce.

5. Ladle the sauce over the meat or pour it into a heated gravy boat.

Poached Swordfish with Lemon-Parsley Sauce

Swordfish steaks are usually cut thicker than most fish fillets, plus they're a firmer fish so it takes longer to poach them. You can speed up the poaching process a little if you remove the steaks from the refrigerator and put them in room-temperature water during the 30 minutes of Step 1.

INGREDIENTS | SERVES 4

1 tablespoon butter

4 thin slices sweet onion

2 cups water

4 (6-ounce) swordfish steaks

Sea salt, to taste

1 large lemon

2 tablespoons extra-virgin olive oil

2 teaspoons fresh lemon juice

¼ teaspoon gluten-free Dijon mustard

Freshly ground white or black pepper, to taste (optional)

1 tablespoon minced fresh flat-leaf parsley

Swordfish Salad

Triple the amount of lemon-parsley sauce and toss ⅔ of it together with 8 cups of salad greens. Arrange 2 cups of greens on each serving plate. Place a hot or chilled swordfish steak over each plate of the dressed greens. Spoon the additional sauce over the fish.

1. Grease the bottom and halfway up the side of the slow cooker with butter. Arrange onion slices over the bottom of the slow cooker, pressing them into the butter so that they stay in place. Pour in water. Cover and cook on high for 30 minutes.

2. Place a swordfish steak over each onion slice. Add salt to taste. Thinly slice lemon; discard the seeds and place the slices over the fish.

3. Cover and cook on high for 45 minutes or until the fish is opaque. Transfer the (well-drained) fish to individual serving plates or to a serving platter.

4. Add oil, lemon juice, mustard, and white or black pepper, if using, to a bowl; whisk to combine. Immediately before serving the swordfish, fold in parsley. Evenly divide the sauce between the swordfish steaks.

Beef Bourguignon

For a complete fine-dining experience, serve Beef Bourguignon over buttered gluten-free noodles with Creamed Carrots (see recipe in Chapter 16).

INGREDIENTS | SERVES 8

8 slices bacon, diced

1 large yellow onion, diced

3 cloves garlic, minced

1 (3-pound) boneless English or chuck roast

16 ounces fresh cremini mushrooms, sliced, divided

2 tablespoons tomato paste

2 cups Beef Broth (see recipe in Chapter 11) or water

4 cups Burgundy wine

½ teaspoon dried thyme

1 dried bay leaf

Salt and freshly ground black pepper, to taste

1 large yellow onion, thinly sliced

½ cup butter, softened (optional)

½ cup gluten-free oat flour (optional)

1. In a large nonstick skillet, fry bacon over medium heat until it renders its fat. Use a slotted spoon to remove the bacon and reserve it for another use. Add diced onion to the skillet and sauté for 5 minutes or until transparent. Stir in garlic; sauté for 30 seconds, and then transfer the onion mixture to a 6-quart slow cooker. Cover the cooker.

2. Trim roast of any fat and cut it into bite-sized pieces; add to the skillet and brown over medium-high heat for 5 minutes. Transfer to the slow cooker. Cover. Add half the sliced mushrooms to the skillet; stir-fry for 5 minutes or until the liquids have evaporated; transfer to the slow cooker and replace the cover.

3. Add tomato paste to the skillet and sauté for 3 minutes or until the tomato paste just begins to brown. Stir in broth or water, scraping the bottom of the pan to loosen any browned bits and work them into the sauce. Remove the pan from the heat and stir in Burgundy, thyme, bay leaf, salt, and pepper; stir to combine. Pour into the slow cooker. Add the remaining mushrooms and sliced onion to the slow cooker. Cover and cook on low for 8 hours. Remove bay leaf before serving.

4. Optional: To thicken the sauce, use a slotted spoon to transfer the meat, cooked onions, and mushrooms to a serving platter; cover and keep warm. In a small bowl, mix together butter and flour to form a paste; whisk in some of the pan liquid a little at a time to thin the paste. Strain out any lumps. Increase the heat of the cooker to high. When the pan liquids begin to bubble around the edges, whisk in the flour mixture. Cook, stirring constantly, for 15 minutes or until the sauce has thickened enough to coat the back of a spoon. Pour over the meat, mushrooms, and onions on the serving platter.

Curried Cauliflower

Heating herbs and spices before adding them to water intensifies the flavor.

INGREDIENTS | SERVES 6

1 tablespoon olive oil
¼ cup finely diced onion
1½ teaspoons gluten-free curry powder
½ teaspoon ground cumin
½ teaspoon ground coriander
1 teaspoon chili powder
1 teaspoon salt
1 cup diced tomatoes
1 cup water
1 large head cauliflower, chopped

1. Heat olive oil in a 4-quart slow cooker set to medium heat. Add onion and cook for 5 minutes.

2. Add curry powder, cumin, coriander, chili powder, salt, and tomatoes and stir until well combined.

3. Add water and cauliflower to the slow cooker and stir until the cauliflower is coated. Cover and cook over low heat for 3 hours.

Bacon and Broccoli Crustless Quiche

This recipe requires a heatproof 1½–2-quart casserole dish that can rest on the cooking rack in your slow cooker.

INGREDIENTS | SERVES 6

Nonstick cooking spray, as needed

2 cups frozen broccoli cuts, thawed

2 cups grated Colby cheese

6 slices cooked bacon

4 large eggs

2 cups whole milk

Salt and freshly ground black pepper, to taste

½ teaspoon gluten-free Dijon mustard

1 tablespoon mayonnaise

1. Treat a casserole dish with nonstick spray. Arrange broccoli cuts over the bottom of the dish, and top with grated cheese. Cut bacon into pieces and sprinkle evenly over the top.

2. Add eggs to a bowl or large measuring cup. Lightly beat the eggs and then stir in the milk, salt, pepper, mustard, and mayonnaise. Pour over the broccoli mixture in the casserole dish.

3. Place the casserole dish onto the cooking rack in the slow cooker. Pour water into the slow cooker so that it comes up and over the cooking rack and about 1" up the sides of the casserole dish. Cover and cook on low for 4 hours.

4. Turn off the slow cooker. Uncover and allow to cool enough so you can lift the casserole dish out of the cooker. Cut the crustless quiche into 6 wedges. Serve warm or at room temperature.

Tarragon Chicken

This rich French dish can stand on its own when served with just a tossed salad and some crusty bread.

INGREDIENTS | SERVES 4

½ cup plus 2 tablespoons gluten-free oat flour

½ teaspoon salt

8 large chicken thighs, skin removed

2 tablespoons butter

2 tablespoons olive oil

1 medium yellow onion, diced

1 cup dry white wine

1 cup Chicken Broth (see recipe in Chapter 11)

½ teaspoon dried tarragon

1 cup heavy cream

Tarragon Chicken Cooking Times

After 4 hours, the chicken will be cooked through. If you want to leave the chicken cooking all day, after 8 hours the meat will fall away from the bone. You can then remove the bones before you stir in the cream.

1. Add ½ cup flour, salt, and chicken thighs to a 1-gallon resealable plastic bag. Close the bag and shake to coat the chicken.

2. Add butter and oil to a large sauté pan and bring to temperature over medium-high heat. Add chicken thighs and brown on each side, about 5 minutes per side.

3. Drain the chicken on paper towels, and then place in the slow cooker. Cover the slow cooker. Set temperature to low.

4. Add onion to the sauté pan and sauté until transparent. Stir in 2 tablespoons flour, and cook the flour until the onion just begins to brown. Slowly pour the wine into the pan, stirring to scrape up the browned bits from the bottom of the pan and into the sauce. Add broth.

5. Cook and stir for 15 minutes or until the sauce is thickened enough to coat the back of a spoon. Stir in tarragon, and then pour the sauce over the chicken in the slow cooker. Cover and cook for 4–8 hours.

6. Pour cream into the slow cooker; cover and cook for an additional 15 minutes or until the cream is heated through. Test for seasoning and add additional salt and tarragon if needed. Serve immediately.

Moroccan Root Vegetables

Moroccan Root Vegetables is good served with couscous, yogurt dipping sauce, and a simple side salad.

INGREDIENTS | SERVES 8

1 pound parsnips, peeled and diced

1 pound turnips, peeled and diced

2 medium onions, chopped

1 pound carrots, peeled and diced

6 dried apricots, chopped

4 pitted prunes, chopped

1 teaspoon ground turmeric

1 teaspoon ground cumin

½ teaspoon ground ginger

½ teaspoon ground cinnamon

¼ teaspoon ground cayenne pepper

1 tablespoon dried parsley

1 tablespoon dried cilantro

2 cups Vegetable Stock (see recipe in Chapter 11)

1 teaspoon salt

1. Add parsnips, turnips, onions, carrots, apricots, prunes, turmeric, cumin, ginger, cinnamon, cayenne pepper, parsley, and cilantro to a 4-quart slow cooker.

2. Pour in stock and salt.

3. Cover and cook on low for 9 hours, or until the vegetables are cooked through.

Applesauce

You'll need about 4 pounds of apples for this size batch of applesauce, or enough to fill the slow cooker ¾ full. The amount of sugar that you use will depend on the sweetness of the apples and your personal taste.

INGREDIENTS | MAKES ABOUT 4 CUPS

12 medium apples
½–1 cup pure cane sugar
Pinch salt
1 tablespoon lemon juice (optional)

Spiced Applesauce

In Step 1, cook on low for 4 hours and then stir in 1 teaspoon ground cinnamon, ½ teaspoon ground cloves, ¼ teaspoon ground ginger, ¼ teaspoon allspice, and a pinch of freshly ground nutmeg. Cover and cook for another hour before proceeding to Step 2. Taste the applesauce after you've added the sugar and increase the amounts of spices if desired.

1. Peel, core, and slice apples. Add to the slow cooker. Cover and cook on low for 5 hours.

2. Stir in sugar and salt. Use an immersion blender to purée the apples. Cover and cook on low for an additional 30 minutes or until the sugar is dissolved.

3. Optional: If the applesauce is too sweet, stir in the lemon juice to help balance the sweetness.

4. Serve warm as an accompaniment to pork chops or over pancakes. For leftovers, cool and store in the refrigerator for 2–3 days, or pour into appropriate covered containers and freeze for up to 3 months.

Cranberry Pear Compote

You can serve this compote warm over gluten-free pound cake or cooled with whipped cream. You can layer the chilled compote in parfait glasses with whipped cream and pieces of pound cake, broken fig-filled cookies, or gluten-free graham cracker crumbs.

INGREDIENTS | SERVES 8

1 cup water
½ cup port or Madeira wine
½ cup granulated sugar
6 allspice berries
4 cardamom pods, crushed
1 cup fresh cranberries
4 large pears

1. Add water, wine, sugar, allspice, and cardamom to a 4-quart slow cooker. Cover and cook on high for 30 minutes or until the liquid is bubbling around the edges. Stir to dissolve the sugar into the liquid.

2. Rinse and drain cranberries. Remove and discard any stems or blemished cranberries. Stir into the liquid in the slow cooker. Cover and cook on high for 30 minutes or until the cranberries pop.

3. Peel, core, and cut pears into quarters. Stir into other ingredients in the slow cooker. Cover and cook on low for 6 hours or on high for 3 hours.

4. Remove and discard the allspice berries and cardamom pods. Serve warm from the slow cooker, or let come to room temperature and pour into a covered container. Refrigerate until chilled.

Fruit Crisp

Serve with ice cream or with a dollop of whipped cream on top.

INGREDIENTS | SERVES 4

6 large peaches
¼ cup granulated sugar
2 teaspoons ground cinnamon
Nonstick cooking spray, as needed
¾ cup rolled oats
¼ cup gluten-free oat flour
½ packed cup brown sugar
6 tablespoons butter
1 cup pecans

Quicker and Easier Fruit Crisp

Fruit crisp is a versatile dessert. You don't have to limit yourself to fresh fruit. If you need to throw together a dessert in a hurry, you can thaw some frozen peaches or open a can of any pie filling and use one of those instead.

1. Peel peaches. Cut in half, remove pits, and slice peaches. Toss together with sugar and cinnamon.

2. Treat a 4-quart slow cooker with nonstick spray. Arrange the peaches over the bottom of the slow cooker.

3. To make the topping, add oats, flour, brown sugar, and butter to a food processor. Pulse until the topping is the consistency of coarse cornmeal. Add pecans and pulse a couple of times to rough-chop the nuts and mix them into the topping.

4. Sprinkle the topping evenly over the fruit in the slow cooker. Cover and cook on high for 2 hours or until the peaches are tender and the topping is crisp. Serve warm or chilled.

Mocha Custard

If you're impatient and indulgent, spoon this custard directly from the slow cooker and use the custard as hot sauce over ice cream. Otherwise, serve chilled according to the recipe instructions.

INGREDIENTS | SERVES 4

¼ cup instant espresso powder

2 tablespoons unsweetened cocoa powder, plus extra for garnish if desired

⅔ cup granulated sugar

Pinch salt

4 cups half-and-half

6 large eggs

½ teaspoon vanilla or maple extract

Nonstick cooking spray, as needed

Whipped cream (optional)

1. Add espresso powder, cocoa powder, sugar, and salt to a blender or food processor. Pulse to mix and remove any lumps.

2. Add half-and-half, eggs, and extract to the blender or food processor. Process until blended.

3. Treat a 4-quart slow cooker with nonstick spray. Pour in the custard mixture. Cover and cook on low for 2½ hours, or until the edges of the custard begin to puff and a knife inserted in the center comes out clean.

4. Remove the crock from the slow cooker; place it on hot pads or a rack. Let the custard stand at room temperature for 1 hour or until cooled.

5. Cover the top of the crock with plastic wrap or the slow cooker lid; refrigerate for 4 hours. Serve spooned into custard cups or your favorite dessert stemware. Top with a dollop of whipped cream dusted with cocoa powder, if desired.

CHAPTER 18

Desserts

Flourless Hazelnut Chocolate Cake

In this melt-in-your-mouth cake, traditional acid reflux–causing
white flour is replaced by nutrient-dense hazelnuts.

INGREDIENTS | SERVES 12

Nonstick cooking spray, as needed

3½ cups ground roasted hazelnuts

1½ cups Splenda No Calorie Sweetener, granulated

2 tablespoons vanilla extract

¾ cup unsweetened cocoa powder

12 egg whites

1. Preheat oven to 350°F. Coat a 10" springform pan with nonstick cooking spray.

2. Mix hazelnuts, Splenda, vanilla, and cocoa in a medium-sized bowl. Beat egg whites in a large glass bowl until stiff. Gently fold egg whites into chocolate-nut mixture.

3. Pour batter into the prepared pan. Bake for 40–50 minutes or until a toothpick inserted into the cake comes out clean.

4. Let cool before serving.

Raspberry Coulis

This is delectable over ice cream, sherbet, or sorbet.

INGREDIENTS | SERVES 6

8 ounces raspberries, gently washed

1 teaspoon lemon juice

Sugar substitute, to taste (start with 1 packet)

Blend all ingredients in a blender. Strain and serve.

Nut-Crusted Key Lime Pie

Nut crusts are versatile and delicious with almost any kind of pie. Although nuts are fattening, they are still good for you—they contain high amounts of fiber and vitamin E.

INGREDIENTS | SERVES 8

Nonstick cooking spray, as needed

1 cup macadamia nuts, pecans, or walnuts, coarsely ground

1 cup graham cracker crumbs

1 stick butter, melted

1 tablespoon dark brown sugar

Rind of ½ medium orange

1½ cups cold water, divided

⅓ cup cornstarch

Juice of 3 medium limes

2 packets unflavored gelatin

2 egg yolks

3 egg whites, beaten stiff

2 tablespoons sugar substitute

1. Preheat oven to 325°F. Prepare a 9" pie pan with non-stick spray.

2. In a food processor or blender, mix nuts, cracker crumbs, butter, brown sugar, and orange rind to the texture of oatmeal.

3. Press the nut mixture into the prepared pan. Bake for 30 minutes, or until crisp and lightly browned. Set aside to cool, then refrigerate.

4. In a blender, mix 1 cup cold water and all remaining ingredients except egg whites and sugar substitute. Add remaining water and pour into a medium saucepan. Whisking constantly, bring to a boil. Cool until almost stiff.

5. Place filling mixture into the well-chilled pie shell. Fold sugar substitute into beaten egg whites and spread over lime filling.

6. Increase oven temperature to 350°F. Bake pie until golden brown.

Baked Stuffed Apples

For breakfast or dessert, baked apples are a delightful, spicy, and warm treat.

INGREDIENTS | SERVES 2

2 large apples, such as Macintosh, Rome, or Granny Smith

2 teaspoons brown sugar

½ teaspoon ground cinnamon

2 teaspoons chopped walnuts

2 teaspoons raisins

2 teaspoons butter

2 tablespoons water

Creamy Additions

The spices in these baked, stuffed apples and the tartness of the apples are both complemented nicely by dairy. You can serve these with a little cream poured over the top or a scoop of vanilla ice cream on the side for added richness.

1. Preheat oven to 350°F. Using a corer, remove the center portions of the apples, being careful not to cut through the bottom of the apple.

2. For each apple, form a cup to hold the apple with a double layer of aluminum foil, going ⅓ of the way up the apple. This will stabilize the apple when baking.

3. Mix together brown sugar, cinnamon, walnuts, and raisins and stuff the mixture into the apples. Top each apple with 1 teaspoon butter. Put 1 tablespoon water into each aluminum foil cup.

4. Bake for 25 minutes, or until the apples are soft when pierced with a fork.

Simple Berry Crumble

Try this recipe with a variety of succulent berries to satisfy your sweet tooth.

INGREDIENTS | SERVES 4

1 (12-ounce) bag frozen berries, or 2 cups fresh berries

¼ cup unsalted butter, softened

3 tablespoons Splenda No Calorie Sweetener, granulated

2 large eggs

1 teaspoon vanilla extract

¼ teaspoon salt

½ teaspoon baking powder

½ cup almond flour

1. Preheat oven to 375°F.

2. Place berries in an 8" × 8" glass baking dish.

3. In a medium mixing bowl, whip butter and Splenda with a fork. Mix in eggs, vanilla, and salt until well blended.

4. In a small bowl, stir together the baking powder and almond flour. Add almond flour mixture to butter and egg mixture and mix well.

5. Spread the batter over the fruit. Bake for 25 minutes, or until golden brown on top.

Gingerbread Pudding Cake

This cake may not be the prettiest cake you'll ever make,
but the warm spices paired with vanilla bean ice cream is excellent.

INGREDIENTS | SERVES 6

Nonstick cooking spray, as needed

½ cup brown rice flour

½ cup arrowroot starch

½ cup granulated sugar

1 teaspoon baking powder

¼ teaspoon baking soda

1¼ teaspoons ground ginger

½ teaspoon ground cinnamon

¾ cup 2% milk

1 large egg

½ cup raisins

2¼ cups water

¾ cup packed cup brown sugar

½ cup butter

1. Grease a 4-quart slow cooker with nonstick cooking spray. In a medium bowl, whisk together flour, arrowroot starch, sugar, baking powder, baking soda, ginger, and cinnamon.

2. Stir milk and egg into dry ingredients. Stir in raisins (batter will be thick). Spread gingerbread batter evenly in the bottom of the prepared cooker.

3. In a medium saucepan, combine water, brown sugar, and butter. Bring to a boil; reduce heat. Boil gently, uncovered, for 2 minutes. Carefully pour sugar mixture over gingerbread batter.

4. Cover and vent lid with a chopstick or the end of a wooden spoon. Cook on high for 2–2½ hours, until the cake is cooked through and a toothpick inserted about ½" into the center comes out clean. (It may not look like it's all the way cooked through.)

5. Remove insert from slow cooker. Let cool for 45–60 minutes to allow "pudding" to set beneath the cake.

6. To serve, spoon warm cake into dessert dishes and spoon pudding sauce over the top.

Creamy Hot Fudge Sauce

Try this sauce over frozen yogurt or ice cream.

INGREDIENTS | MAKES 2 CUPS

12 ounces evaporated milk

10 ounces semisweet or bittersweet chocolate chips

1 teaspoon vanilla extract

½ teaspoon butter

⅛ teaspoon salt

1. Place all ingredients in a 1½–2-quart slow cooker. Cook on low, stirring occasionally, for 2 hours. The sauce will thicken as it cools.

2. Refrigerate leftovers. Reheat in the slow cooker for 1 hour on high or on the stovetop until warmed through, about 10 minutes.

Frozen Bananas Dipped in Chocolate

Kids love these—and so do lots of grownups. They're a snap to make, and you can involve older kids in the dipping.

INGREDIENTS | SERVES 10

10 medium bananas
10 Popsicle sticks
Nonstick cooking spray, as needed
1 pound semisweet chocolate
Pinch salt
1 teaspoon vanilla extract

1. Peel bananas and insert Popsicle sticks. Place bananas on a baking sheet you have prepared with nonstick spray and freeze.

2. Just before serving, melt chocolate in a large saucepan. Add salt and vanilla. Let cool until warm, but don't let harden.

3. Dip frozen bananas into chocolate and place on waxed paper. The frozen bananas will harden the chocolate, and they're ready to eat right away.

Dark Chocolate, Walnut, and Hazelnut Torte

This is exceedingly rich and delicious. Fresh whipped cream or a few fresh raspberries on the side make an excellent garnish.

INGREDIENTS | SERVES 14

1 pound bittersweet chocolate, chopped

1 cup unsalted butter, cut into pieces

¼ cup unsweetened cocoa powder

¼ cup hazelnut liqueur

½ teaspoon vanilla extract

5 large eggs

2 teaspoons grated orange zest

1 cup hazelnuts, toasted, skinned, and ground

1 cup walnuts, toasted and ground

½ cup confectioners' sugar

Vanilla

Whatever you do, don't use imitation vanilla extract—the pure stuff is a bit more expensive, but it tastes so much better it's worth it. Imitation vanilla extract may give food a slight chemical flavor. You can use vanilla beans to make flavored sugar: Simply slit open a bean and place it in a jar with 2 cups granulated sugar, seal, and let sit for 1 week.

1. Preheat oven to 350°F. Grease a 9" cake pan and line with parchment paper.

2. In the top of a double boiler, heat chocolate and butter until chocolate melts. Remove from heat and stir.

3. Add cocoa powder, liqueur, vanilla, eggs, and orange zest, mixing well.

4. Add hazelnuts and walnuts and mix. Pour batter into the prepared cake pan. Bake until the cake is barely set, about 25–30 minutes.

5. Cool in the pan for 20 minutes. Remove from pan and place on a rack.

6. Cool completely and sprinkle with confectioners' sugar.

Blueberry-Peach Cobbler

This smells and tastes like an August dessert; however, if you blanch and freeze your peaches and buy frozen blueberries, you can reminisce over a past August in January.

INGREDIENTS | SERVES 10

6 ripe peaches, blanched in boiling water, skinned, pitted, and sliced

½ cup fresh lemon juice

1 cup granulated sugar, divided

1 pint blueberries, rinsed and picked over, stems removed

½ cup unsalted butter, melted

½ teaspoon salt

1½ cups rice flour or quinoa flour

1 tablespoon baking powder

1 cup buttermilk

1. Preheat oven to 375°F. Prepare a 9" × 13" baking dish with nonstick spray.

2. Add peaches to a large bowl and sprinkle with lemon juice and ½ cup sugar. Add blueberries and mix well.

3. Spread the peaches and blueberries on the bottom of the prepared pan. Pour melted butter into a large bowl. Add remaining ½ cup su0gar and salt and whisk in flour and baking powder. Add buttermilk and stir; don't worry about lumps.

4. Drop the batter by tablespoonsful over the fruit. Bake for 35–40 minutes. Cool for 25 minutes. Serve with vanilla ice cream or whipped cream.

Dark Chocolate–Dipped Strawberries

This crowd-pleaser is always delicious and is good to make in advance.
Make sure to purchase the best strawberries you can find.

INGREDIENTS | MAKES 36 BERRIES

36 very large strawberries with long stems

14 ounces dark chocolate (70 percent cocoa)

2 tablespoons heavy cream

A Valentine's Treat

One of the most popular Valentine's Day gifts is chocolate-dipped strawberries, with their bloom of red along with creamy or dark chocolate. Surprise your loved one with a homemade rendition that will melt her heart.

1. Rinse berries and let dry on paper towels.

2. Melt chocolate in a double boiler over simmering water. Remove from heat and stir in heavy cream.

3. Carefully dip strawberries, 1 at a time, in chocolate. Store in a cool place, or if made more than 5 hours ahead of time, store in the refrigerator.

CHAPTER 19

Gluten-Free Breads

Classic Sandwich Bread

This easy and delicious gluten-free yeast bread recipe uses as few ingredients as possible.

INGREDIENTS | YIELDS 1 (8 ½" × 4 ½") LOAF OF GLUTEN-FREE BREAD

1 cup brown rice flour

1 cup arrowroot starch or tapioca starch

3 tablespoons ground flaxseeds

3 tablespoons gluten-free rolled oats

½ teaspoon salt

1½ teaspoons xanthan gum

2 teaspoons SAF-Instant Yeast, Red Star Quick-Rise or Bread Machine Yeast, or Fleischmann's Bread Machine Yeast

3 tablespoons sugar or honey

2 large eggs, room temperature

1 cup plus 2 tablespoons milk or almond milk, heated to 110°F

2 tablespoons olive oil

Proofing Basics

In many bread recipes you need to "proof" the yeast by mixing it with warm water or milk and a little sugar. This activates the yeast, or helps it to start digesting the sugar to grow and create air bubbles that help the bread dough rise. Most of the yeast bread recipes in this chapter call for instant yeast (also called rapid-rise or bread-machine yeast), as opposed to active dry or fresh yeast—and instant yeast does not need to be proofed to start working. The yeast will start working as soon as it's mixed into the dry ingredients and introduced to warm water.

1. In a large bowl whisk together brown rice flour, arrowroot starch, ground flaxseeds, oats, salt, xanthan gum, yeast, and sugar. In a smaller bowl whisk together eggs, milk, and olive oil.

2. Pour wet ingredients into dry ingredients. Stir with a wooden spoon or a fork for several minutes until batter resembles a thick cake batter. First it will look like biscuit dough, but after a few minutes it will appear thick and sticky.

3. Line an 8½" × 4½" metal or glass loaf pan with parchment paper or spritz generously with nonstick cooking spray. Pour bread dough into the pan. Using a spatula that's been dipped in water or spritzed with oil or nonstick cooking spray, spread the dough evenly in the pan. Continue to use the spatula to smooth out the top of the dough.

4. Cover the pan with a tea towel or cover loosely with plastic wrap that has been spritzed with nonstick spray or olive oil (so it will not stick to the dough). Allow dough to rise in a warm space for 1–2 hours until doubled in size. The top of the loaf should rise about 1" above the lip of the pan.

5. Once your dough has doubled, preheat the oven to 425°F. Remove the covering from the loaf and bake for 25–35 minutes. If the bread begins to brown more than desired, place a sheet of foil over the loaf and continue baking. The bread will be done when the internal temperature is between 190°F–200°F, when tested with a food thermometer. Allow bread to cool completely on a wire rack for 2–3 hours before slicing. If you slice the bread when it is still hot, it may lose its shape and fall.

6. Bread will keep on the counter in a zip-top plastic bag for 2–3 days. After 3 days, slice and freeze the remaining loaf.

Focaccia

This chewy and crunchy bread would also make an outstanding deep-dish pizza crust.

INGREDIENTS | YIELDS 12–16 SLICES, DEPENDING ON SIZE

1½ cups brown rice flour

½ cup sorghum flour

2 cups arrowroot starch or tapioca starch

⅔ cup blanched almond flour or nonfat dry milk powder

1 tablespoon xanthan gum

2 teaspoons SAF-Instant Yeast, Red Star Quick-Rise or Bread Machine Yeast, or Fleischmann's Bread Machine Yeast

1 teaspoon salt

1½ cups water, heated to 110°F

3 tablespoons olive oil

4 large egg whites, room temperature

1 clove garlic, finely minced

Fresh herbs, finely chopped (such as rosemary, oregano, or thyme)

Olive oil for spreading dough

Chopped and seeded kalamata olives and Roma tomatoes (optional)

Should You Invest in a Heavy-Duty Stand Mixer?

Nearly all the recipes in this chapter can be made much easier and faster in a heavy-duty stand mixer. This recipe in particular makes a very thick dough and it can be hard to mix just using your hands and a fork. If you have a stand mixer, mix this dough using the dough hook attachment. Allow it to work the dough for 5–6 minutes if you have time, then bake as directed. If you have arthritis or other joint problems, or if you plan on baking every day or several times a week, a stand mixer may be a good investment.

1. Line a 9" × 14" baking dish with parchment paper and grease with nonstick cooking spray or olive oil.

2. In a large bowl whisk together brown rice flour, sorghum flour, arrowroot starch or tapioca starch, almond flour or milk powder, xanthan gum, yeast, and salt. In another bowl whisk together water, olive oil, and egg whites. Pour wet ingredients into dry ingredients and stir together thoroughly into a stiff dough. Continue to mix as much as you can (it is a very stiff dough) for an additional 3–4 minutes.

3. Transfer the dough to baking dish. Drizzle the dough with a little olive oil and then evenly spread dough over the entire baking dish. Cover the dough lightly with plastic wrap and allow to rise in a warm place for about 35 minutes.

4. When ready to bake, preheat oven to 400°F. Gently poke the dough all over with your fingers so small wells appear in the dough. Drizzle with additional olive oil and sprinkle on the minced garlic and any of the additional toppings you like.

5. Bake for 15–20 minutes until focaccia is golden-brown and crispy. Allow to cool for 10 minutes, then slice into squares and serve.

Challah

This challah bread is lightly sweetened and moist. Your family will never know it's gluten-free.

INGREDIENTS | YIELDS 1 (1 ½-POUND) LOAF OF BREAD

2 cups brown rice flour

1¾ cups arrowroot starch or tapioca starch

¼ cup sugar

1 teaspoon salt

2½ teaspoons xanthan gum

2½ teaspoons SAF-Instant Yeast, Red Star Quick-Rise or Bread Machine Yeast, or Fleischmann's Bread Machine Yeast

4 large eggs, room temperature

1⅔ cups water, heated to 110°F

1 teaspoon apple cider vinegar

4 tablespoons melted butter

Sesame seeds (optional)

1. In a large bowl whisk together brown rice flour, arrowroot starch or tapioca starch, sugar, salt, xanthan gum, and yeast. In a smaller bowl whisk together the eggs, water, vinegar, and butter.

2. Pour wet ingredients into dry ingredients. Stir with a wooden spoon or a fork for several minutes until batter resembles a thick cake batter. First it will look like biscuit dough, but after a few minutes it will appear thick and sticky.

3. Line a 1½-pound loaf pan (10" × 5") with parchment paper or spritz generously with nonstick cooking spray. Pour bread dough into the pan. Using a spatula that's been dipped in water or spritzed with oil or nonstick cooking spray, spread the dough evenly in the pan. Continue to use the spatula to smooth the top of the dough.

4. Cover the pan with a tea towel or cover loosely with plastic wrap that has been spritzed with nonstick spray or olive oil (so it will not stick to the dough). Allow the dough to rise in a warm space for 1–2 hours until doubled in size. The top of the loaf should rise about 1" above the lip of the pan.

5. Once dough has doubled, preheat the oven to 425°F. Remove the covering from the loaf and, if desired, sprinkle dough with sesame seeds. Bake for 35–45 minutes. If the bread begins to brown more than desired, place a sheet of foil over the loaf and continue baking.

6. Bread will be done when the internal temperature is 190°F–200°F when tested with a food thermometer. Allow bread to cool completely on a wire rack for 2–3 hours before slicing. If the bread is sliced when it is still hot, it may lose its shape and fall.

7. Bread will keep on the counter in a zip-top plastic bag for 2–3 days. After 3 days, slice and freeze the remaining loaf.

French Bread

This recipe makes two loaves of tasty, crusty French bread. Eat one with your meal and freeze the extra loaf and voilà, you have instant French bread that can be heated in 15–20 minutes in a preheated oven.

INGREDIENTS | YIELDS 2 LOAVES

1 cup arrowroot starch or tapioca starch

2 cups brown rice flour

½ teaspoon sea salt

1 tablespoon xanthan gum

1½ tablespoons SAF-Instant Yeast, Red Star Quick-Rise or Bread Machine Yeast, or Fleischmann's Bread Machine Yeast

2 tablespoons sugar

3 large egg whites

1½ cups water, heated to 110°F

2 tablespoons olive oil

1 teaspoon apple cider vinegar

1 large egg white, lightly beaten with 1 tablespoon water

1. In a large bowl whisk together arrowroot starch, brown rice flour, salt, xanthan gum, yeast, and sugar. In a smaller bowl whisk together the egg whites, water, olive oil, and vinegar.

2. Pour wet ingredients into dry ingredients. Stir with a wooden spoon for several minutes until batter resembles a thick cake batter. First it will look like biscuit dough, but after a few minutes it will appear thick and sticky.

3. Line a French bread pan or baguette pan with parchment paper or spritz generously with nonstick cooking spray. Divide the dough in half and pour into the pan. Shape two long loaves using a spatula that's been dipped in water or spritzed with oil or nonstick cooking spray. Spread the dough evenly in the pan. Continue to use the spatula to smooth the top and sides of the dough. Using a sharp knife, make 3–4 cuts about ¼" deep across the top of each loaf.

4. Cover the pan with a tea towel or cover loosely with plastic wrap that has been spritzed with nonstick spray or olive oil (so it will not stick to the dough). Allow the dough to rise in a warm space for 1–2 hours until it's doubled in size.

5. Once dough has doubled, preheat the oven to 350°F. Remove the covering from the loaf, brush each loaf gently with the egg white and water mixture, and bake for 35 minutes. After 35 minutes, place a sheet of foil over the loaf and continue baking for an additional 20 minutes. Allow bread to cool completely on a wire rack for 30 minutes to 1 hour before slicing.

6. Bread will keep on the counter in a zip-top plastic bag for 2–3 days. After 3 days, slice and freeze the remaining loaf.

Italian Breadsticks

This recipe uses psyllium husks instead of gums to give bread structure and texture, without eggs.

INGREDIENTS | YIELDS 20–30 BREADSTICKS

2 cups brown rice flour

1⅓ cups arrowroot starch or tapioca starch

2¼ teaspoons SAF-Instant Yeast, Red Star Quick-Rise or Bread Machine Yeast, or Fleischmann's Bread Machine Yeast

3 tablespoons psyllium seed husks

2 teaspoons sea salt

½ teaspoon baking soda

¼ cup olive oil

2 tablespoons coconut palm sugar or vegan sugar

2 tablespoons unsweetened applesauce

2⅓ cups warm water

2 tablespoons almond milk

Sesame seeds (optional)

1. Preheat oven to 350°F. Line a large cookie sheet with parchment paper and then grease with nonstick cooking spray or light-tasting olive oil.

2. In a large bowl whisk together brown rice flour, arrowroot starch, yeast, psyllium husks, salt, and baking soda. Make a well in the center of the dry ingredients and add olive oil, sugar, applesauce, and warm water. Mix together until you have a pancake-like batter. Batter will be thinner than a regular gluten-free bread dough.

3. Cover dough and let it very slowly rise overnight in the refrigerator, or you can cover it and place it on the counter in a warm place to double in size, about 1–2 hours.

4. When the dough has risen and you are ready to make breadsticks, preheat oven to 450°F. This batter makes a lot of breadsticks, so feel free to only use half the dough and place the rest in the fridge for the next day.

5. Make a breadstick by scooping out 2–4 tablespoons of dough and rolling it in a ball on a brown rice–floured surface. Gently roll the dough out like a snake in a breadstick form. Place the dough 2" apart on the cookie sheet. Cover lightly and allow the dough to rest for 30 minutes before baking. This will allow the breadsticks to rise a bit more.

6. When the breadsticks are ready to bake, brush them lightly with almond milk and sprinkle with sesame seeds, if desired. For soft breadsticks, bake for 10–15 minutes. For more crispy breadsticks, bake for 25–30 minutes. Allow breadsticks to cool for 5 minutes before serving. Store bread in an airtight container on the counter for up to 1 week. Baked breadsticks will also freeze for up to 2 months.

Irish Soda Bread

Serve this biscuit-like bread on St. Patrick's Day or any cool day with a big bowl of hot soup or stew.

INGREDIENTS | YIELDS 1 (8" OR 9") ROUND LOAF

Brown rice flour, for sprinkling
1½ cups sorghum flour
½ cup arrowroot or tapioca starch
2 tablespoons sugar
1 teaspoon baking soda
1½ teaspoons baking powder
1 teaspoon sea salt
1½ teaspoons xanthan gum
6 tablespoons cold butter or Spectrum Palm Shortening
¾ cup buttermilk or non-dairy milk mixed with 1 teaspoon apple cider vinegar or lemon juice
2 large eggs
1 cup currants or raisins

1. Preheat oven to 375°F. Line a baking sheet with parchment paper, and sprinkle with brown rice flour. Set aside.

2. In the bowl of a food processor, combine sorghum flour, arrowroot starch or tapioca starch, sugar, baking soda, baking powder, salt, and xanthan gum. Pulse to combine ingredients. (If you don't have a food processor, combine all dry ingredients in a medium-sized mixing bowl and whisk together well.)

3. Add the butter or shortening and pulse until the butter is the size of peas. Or, use a pastry blender to cut the butter into the dry ingredients, working quickly because you want the butter to stay cold.

4. Add the buttermilk and eggs, and run the food processor until the dough comes together in a sticky ball. (Alternately, you can use a wooden spoon and stir until the dough comes together.) Stir in the raisins or currants.

5. Turn dough out onto baking sheet and flour your hands with more brown rice flour. Working quickly, pat the dough down into a large 8" or 9" circle. With a sharp knife, cut an "X" about ¼" deep into the center of the loaf. Gently brush the top of the loaf with additional buttermilk or non-dairy milk.

6. Bake for 30 minutes, or until the loaf is golden-brown and crispy on top. Allow to cool for 25–30 minutes on a cooling rack before slicing into 8 triangles and serving. Store any remaining bread in an airtight container on the counter for 2–3 days.

English Muffins

There's something incredibly comforting about this cornmeal-crusted, tender bread with big air pockets that soak up lots of butter and jam. Some English muffins are cooked on the stovetop, but these are baked, and are a little less work.

INGREDIENTS | SERVES 8

Gluten-free coarse cornmeal, for sprinkling
½ cup sorghum flour
¼ cup brown rice flour
¾ cup arrowroot starch
1 teaspoon xanthan gum
½ teaspoon salt
1 tablespoon sugar
2 teaspoons rapid-rise yeast
1 teaspoon olive oil
¾ cup plus 1 tablespoon hot water

Make Your Own English Muffin Rings

You can buy metal rings to bake English muffins in, or you can make your own. Simply fold sheets of foil into 1"-strips and staple them into a circle about the size of a tuna can. You can also use the metal rings from wide-mouth canning jars. Just place them top-side down on the baking sheet and add the dough.

1. Line a baking sheet with parchment paper and place 6 to 8 English muffin rings or foil rings on the parchment. Generously sprinkle cornmeal in the bottoms of the rings.

2. In a large bowl whisk together sorghum flour, brown rice flour, arrowroot starch, xanthan gum, salt, sugar, and yeast. Make a well in the center of the ingredients and add the olive oil and water. Stir together into a thick batter.

3. Divide the dough evenly between the English muffin rings. Smooth muffin tops by wetting your finger with water and then running your finger gently over the top of each muffin. Generously sprinkle additional cornmeal on top of each muffin. Loosely cover muffins with plastic wrap and set in a warm place to rise for 30–40 minutes.

4. Once the muffins have doubled in size, preheat oven to 375°F. Bake muffins for 15–20 minutes until golden-brown. Flip over the muffins after 8–9 minutes if you want them evenly browned on both sides.

5. Remove the muffins from the rings and allow them to cool for 10–15 minutes before eating. Break muffins apart with a fork to get the nooks and crannies of a traditional English muffin. These muffins are delicious toasted! Muffins are best on the first day. Freeze any remaining muffins for up to 1 month.

Bagels

This recipe makes four jumbo-sized bagels or eight smaller ones. To freeze, wrap them in plastic wrap and put them in a zip-top plastic bag before putting them in the freezer.

INGREDIENTS | SERVES 4

1 cup brown rice flour
½ cup sorghum flour
1 cup arrowroot starch
½ cup ground flaxseeds
1 tablespoon xanthan gum
1½ teaspoons salt
1 tablespoon rapid-rise yeast

2 tablespoons agave nectar or honey
1 teaspoon apple cider vinegar
2 tablespoons oil
1¼ cups warm water
2 teaspoons vegetable shortening, to grease your hands to form the bagels
1 tablespoon molasses
Sesame seeds, flaxseeds, chia seeds, onion flakes, garlic granules, poppy seeds, or coarse salt (optional)

1. Line a baking sheet with parchment paper.

2. In the bowl of a stand mixer, mix all the dry ingredients together until well blended.

3. In a small bowl, whisk together agave nectar or honey, vinegar, oil, and water.

4. With the mixer slowly running, pour in the wet ingredients. Then mix on medium speed for 3 minutes.

5. Grease your hands with the vegetable shortening. Take a quarter of the dough and form it into a bagel shape, using your finger to create a large hole in the center of the bagel. Place the formed bagels on the baking sheet. Give them plenty of space as they will grow a lot as they rise. Repeat to create 4 large bagels.

6. Place the baking sheet in a warm, draft-free place, and allow bagels to rise for 35–40 minutes, or until they are nearly doubled in size.

7. While the bagels are rising, fill a large pot three-quarters full with water. Bring to a rolling boil and add the molasses to the water. (The molasses will create a nice chewy outside to the bagel.)

8. Preheat the oven to 400°F.

9. When the bagels have finished rising, gently place one at a time in the boiling water. Boil on one side for 30 seconds, flip, and boil for another 30 seconds. Remove bagels from water with a slotted spoon, and place on a cooling rack that has been placed over another baking sheet, allowing the water to drip off.

10. Place boiled bagels back on the baking sheet. At this time, you can sprinkle the tops with whatever toppings you desire.

11. Bake the bagels for 20–25 minutes, or until they are golden-brown. Remove from oven, and allow to cool on a cooling rack for 10 minutes before eating. You can eat the bagels warm, or allow them to cool completely before storing in a zip-top plastic bag.

Lemon Poppy Seed Bread

This classic poppy seed loaf is a delicious bread to serve at a spring or Easter luncheon.

INGREDIENTS | SERVES 8

1½ cups brown rice flour

1 cup arrowroot starch

½ teaspoon xanthan gum

½ teaspoon sea salt

1 tablespoon baking powder

¾ cup sugar

3 tablespoons poppy seeds

¼ cup unsweetened applesauce

¼ cup light-tasting olive oil or canola oil

¼ cup fresh lemon juice (about 1 large lemon)

2 tablespoons fresh lemon zest

2 large eggs

¾ cup almond milk

1. Preheat oven to 350°F. Line a 9" × 5" loaf pan with parchment paper and grease with nonstick cooking spray.

2. In a large bowl whisk together brown rice flour, arrowroot starch, xanthan gum, salt, baking powder, sugar, and poppy seeds. In a smaller bowl mix together applesauce, olive oil, lemon juice, lemon zest, eggs, and almond milk. Pour wet ingredients into dry ingredients and stir thoroughly to combine.

3. Pour batter into loaf pan. Bake for 55–65 minutes until a toothpick inserted in the middle comes out clean and top is golden-brown. Allow to cool for 20–30 minutes on a wire rack before slicing.

4. Wrap leftover slices individually in plastic wrap, place in an airtight zip-top plastic bag, and freeze for up to 1 month.

Spiced Apple Bread

Applesauce and fresh apple combine in this delicious recipe to make a quick bread that's perfect for a snack or after-school treat.

INGREDIENTS | SERVES 8

1 cup sorghum flour

¾ cup arrowroot starch

1 teaspoon xanthan gum

¼ teaspoon salt

1 teaspoon ground cinnamon

¼ teaspoon ground nutmeg

⅛ teaspoon ground allspice

⅛ teaspoon ground cardamom

1 teaspoon baking powder

½ teaspoon baking soda

1 cup brown sugar

2 large eggs

2 tablespoons oil

1 teaspoon vanilla

½ cup unsweetened applesauce

1 cup of your favorite apple, peeled and grated

½ cup dried currants (optional)

1. Preheat oven to 350°F. Spray a 9" × 5" loaf pan with nonstick cooking spray and set aside.

2. In a large bowl, combine sorghum flour, arrowroot starch, xanthan gum, salt, cinnamon, nutmeg, allspice, cardamom, baking powder, and baking soda; mix well.

3. In a medium bowl, combine brown sugar, eggs, oil, vanilla, applesauce, apple, and currants, if using; mix well. Stir into dry ingredients just until mixed. Pour into prepared pan.

4. Bake for 50–55 minutes, or until deep golden-brown and a toothpick inserted in the center comes out clean. Let cool in pan for 5 minutes; remove to wire rack to cool completely.

Brown Sugar

Brown sugar can dry out quickly if kept in its original packaging. To make it last longer, buy a brown-sugar disk, a small pottery disk soaked in water. Pack the brown sugar into an airtight container and top with the disk. Make sure the cover is fastened securely. Store in a cool, dark place.

Spiced Holiday Pumpkin Bread

This lovely loaf of fresh pumpkin bread with dried cranberries and toasted pecans makes a beautiful gift for the holidays.

INGREDIENTS | YIELDS 2 MEDIUM LOAVES

⅔ cup arrowroot starch

⅔ cup brown rice flour

⅔ sorghum flour

½ teaspoon xanthan gum

¾ cup coconut palm sugar or vegan sugar

1¼ teaspoons baking powder

1 teaspoon baking soda

2 teaspoons ground cinnamon

½ teaspoon ground cloves

½ teaspoon ginger

¼ teaspoon salt

1¼ cups plain pumpkin purée

¾ cup light-tasting olive oil or canola oil

½ teaspoon apple cider vinegar

½ cup dried cranberries

½ cup chopped, toasted pecans

1. Preheat oven to 350°F. Line 2 (7½" × 3½") loaf pans with parchment paper and then grease with nonstick cooking spray or light-tasting olive oil.

2. In a large bowl whisk together arrowroot starch, brown rice flour, sorghum flour, xanthan gum, sugar, baking powder, baking soda, spices, and salt.

3. In a medium bowl whisk together the pumpkin purée, olive oil, and vinegar. Pour wet ingredients into dry ingredients and mix to combine. Fold in the cranberries and chopped pecans.

4. Divide batter into loaf pans. Smooth tops of loaves with a wet spatula, if desired. Bake for 35–40 minutes until top of bread is golden-brown and a toothpick inserted in the middle comes out clean.

5. Allow bread to cool for 5–10 minutes in the pan before turning out onto a wire rack to cool completely for 1–2 hours. Slice the bread and serve with vegan butter and jam. Store remaining bread in an airtight container on the counter for up to 2 days. Freeze remaining bread for up to 2 months.

Classic Banana Walnut Bread

This bread is sweetened only with bananas. Add up to ¼ cup honey or coconut palm sugar if you prefer your bread a bit sweeter.

INGREDIENTS | YIELDS 1 (8½" × 4½") LOAF

2¼ cups blanched almond flour

¾ cup arrowroot starch or tapioca starch

¼ teaspoon sea salt

1¼ teaspoons baking soda

2 tablespoons melted butter or coconut oil

½ teaspoon apple cider vinegar

3 large eggs

2 cups mashed bananas (about 4 medium)

½ cup chopped walnuts

1. Preheat oven to 350°F. Heavily grease an 8½" × 4½" loaf pan with nonstick cooking spray or olive oil.

2. In a large bowl whisk together the almond flour, arrowroot starch, sea salt, and baking soda. Make a well in the center of the dry ingredients and add butter, vinegar, eggs, and bananas. Mix the wet ingredients into the dry ingredients until you have a thick batter. Fold chopped walnuts into the batter.

3. Pour batter into the greased loaf pan. Smooth the top of the loaf with a spatula dipped in water.

4. Bake for 40–50 minutes until a toothpick inserted in the center of the loaf comes out clean and the top of the bread is golden-brown. Allow to cool in pan for 10 minutes, then place loaf on a wire rack to cool completely. Slice and serve.

Savory Popovers

Popovers are sort of a cross between muffins and pancakes, in a baked form. This savory bread is super easy to make and pretty when taken right from the oven to the table for dinner.

INGREDIENTS | SERVES 6

4 large eggs, room temperature
½ cup almond milk
½ teaspoon sea salt
¼ teaspoon baking soda
2 tablespoons coconut flour

1. Preheat oven to 400°F. Place a muffin tin in the oven while it's preheating to get it very hot.

2. In a large bowl whisk eggs, milk, salt, baking soda and coconut flour, just until bubbly. You don't want to break up the protein in the eggs too much.

3. When the oven has reached the correct temperature, carefully remove the muffin tin with oven mitts. Grease the muffin pan with nonstick cooking spray or brush with olive oil. Fill pan ⅔ full with batter. Place in oven immediately and bake for a full 25 minutes without opening the oven door.

4. Remove pan from oven after 25 minutes and prick the popovers with a sharp knife in the middle to allow the steam to escape. Allow popovers to cool for about 5 minutes and then serve hot with butter or coconut oil and jam.

Flaky Crescent Rolls

This versatile almond flour pastry makes delicious crescent rolls, pie crusts, or personal-size sweet hand pies.

INGREDIENTS | SERVES 10

3 cups blanched almond flour

¼ teaspoon baking soda

½ teaspoon sea salt

4 tablespoons cold butter (cut into cubes), or chilled coconut oil

1 teaspoon honey

2 large eggs

Apple Spice Hand Pies

In a medium bowl mix together 3 peeled, cored, and diced apples; ½ teaspoon cinnamon; ¼ teaspoon nutmeg; and ⅓ cup brown sugar. Mix and roll out pastry as directed. Cut pastry into 4"–6" circles using a cookie cutter. Place 2 tablespoons apple filling on one side of each circle, leaving ½". Fold other half of dough over filling and crimp edges closed with a fork. Brush a little melted butter or coconut oil on top of each pie and sprinkle with cinnamon and sugar. Bake 15–20 minutes until pies are golden-brown. Allow to cool 10–15 minutes before eating.

1. Preheat oven to 400°F. Line a large cookie sheet with parchment paper and set aside.

2. In a large bowl whisk together almond flour, baking soda, and salt. Cut in butter or coconut oil with a pastry blender, until it resembles small peas throughout mixture. Make a well in the center of the dry ingredients and add the honey and eggs. Stir the wet ingredients into the dry ingredients until you have a stiff dough.

3. Shape dough into two large balls. Refrigerate the balls 10–15 minutes before using. Sprinkle additional blanched almond flour onto parchment paper or plastic wrap to help keep the dough from sticking. Place the dough on floured surface. Top with a sheet of parchment paper or plastic wrap and roll out into a 12" circle. Using a pizza cutter, cut into 8 triangles.

4. Roll up triangles starting from the wide end to the point, so they look like crescent rolls. Place each roll about 2" apart on baking sheet. If desired, brush rolls with melted butter or coconut oil.

5. Bake for 12–15 minutes until golden-brown and slightly puffy.

APPENDIX A

Sample Menu Plans

Week 1:

Sunday
Breakfast: Huevos Rancheros (Chapter 16)
Lunch: Veggie Burger Sliders (Chapter 8)
Dinner: Hearty Pot Roast with Creamed Carrots (Chapters 9 and 16)
Dessert: Flourless Hazelnut Chocolate Cake (Chapter 18)
Snack: Stuffed Cherry Tomatoes (Chapter 13)

Monday
Breakfast: Leftover Huevos Rancheros and 1 cup Spicy Melon Juice (Chapter 15)
Lunch: BLT Salad with Turkey and Avocado (Chapter 12)
Dinner: Lemon Chicken with Baked Stuffed Artichokes (Chapters 9 and 10)
Dessert: Leftover Flourless Hazelnut Chocolate Cake
Snack: Pumpkin Spice Smoothie (Chapter 14)

Tuesday
Breakfast: Irish Oatmeal and Poached Fruit (Chapter 7)
Lunch: Thanksgiving Wraps (Chapter 8)
Dinner: Spinach, Sausage, and Bean Soup (Chapter 11)
Dessert: Dark Chocolate–Dipped Strawberries (Chapter 18)
Snack: Spicy Guacamole (Chapter 13) with 1 cup sliced bell pepper

Wednesday
Breakfast: Pineapple Delight Smoothie (Chapter 14)
Lunch: Shrimp and Blood Orange Salad (Chapter 12)
Dinner: Almond Flour Chicken Pot Pie (Chapter 9)
Dessert: Frozen Bananas Dipped in Chocolate (Chapter 18)
Snack: Leftover Spinach, Sausage, and Bean Soup

Thursday
Breakfast: Spinach and Gorgonzola Egg-White Omelet (Chapter 7)
Lunch: Lentil Soup with Winter Vegetables (Chapter 10)
Dinner: Spicy Mixed Meatballs (Chapter 9) with jarred marinara, served over baked spaghetti squash
Dessert: Creamy Hot Fudge Sauce (Chapter 18) drizzled over 1 cup fruit of choice
Snack: Beet and Fruit Smoothie (Chapter 14)

Friday
Breakfast: Sweet Potato Pancakes (Chapter 7)
Lunch: Leftover Lentil Soup with Winter Vegetables
Dinner: Sirloin Steak with Tomato Salad (Chapter 9)
Dessert: Mocha Custard (Chapter 17)
Snack: Deviled Eggs with Capers (Chapter 13)

Saturday
Breakfast: Bacon and Broccoli Crustless Quiche (Chapter 17)
Lunch: Asian Sesame Lettuce Wraps (Chapter 8)
Dinner: Spiced Pumpkin Soup with Garlic and Cheddar Biscuits (Chapters 11 and 10)
Dessert: Leftover Mocha Custard
Snack: Savory Green Smoothie (Chapter 14)

Week 2:

Sunday
Breakfast: Tomato, Bell Pepper, and Feta Frittata (Chapter 7)
Lunch: Grilled Portobello Mushrooms with Lentil Salad (Chapters 9 and 10)
Dinner: Pork Steaks in Apple and Prune Sauce (Chapter 17)
Dessert: Gingerbread Pudding Cake (Chapter 18)
Snack: Berry Almond Scones (Chapter 7)

Monday
Breakfast: Corn Crepes (Chapter 7) with 1 cup fruit of your choice
Lunch: Leftover Tomato, Bell Pepper, and Feta Frittata topped with ½ cup arugula
Dinner: Hearty Lamb Stew (Chapter 11)
Dessert: Leftover Gingerbread Pudding Cake
Snack: 1 cup Pear Pineapple Juice (Chapter 15) and 1 medium banana

Tuesday
Breakfast: Leftover Berry Almond Scones
Lunch: Leftover Hearty Lamb Stew
Dinner: Grilled Eggplant and Pepper Salad (Chapter 12)
Dessert: Raspberry Coulis (Chapter 18) served over ½ cup vanilla ice cream
Snack: Cocoa Banana Smoothie (Chapter 14)

Wednesday
Breakfast: 1 cup low-fat Greek Yogurt drizzled with 2 tablespoons leftover Raspberry Coulis
Lunch: Fig and Parmesan Curl Salad (Chapter 12)
Dinner: Bean and Vegetable Chili (Chapter 10)
Dessert: Blueberry-Peach Cobbler (Chapter 18)
Snack: Sliced cucumber with Mango Salsa (Chapter 13)

Thursday
Breakfast: Mega Melon Smoothie (Chapter 14)
Lunch: Leftover Bean and Vegetable Chili
Dinner: Grilled chicken breast with Honey-Orange Beets (Chapter 16)
Dessert: Leftover Blueberry-Peach Cobbler
Snack: Rosemary Basil Crackers (Chapter 13)

Friday
Breakfast: Blueberry Pancakes (Chapter 7)
Lunch: Shrimp and Lobster Salad (Chapter 8)
Dinner: Moroccan Chicken Tagine (Chapter 9)
Dessert: Fruit Crisp (Chapter 17)
Snack: Stuffed Zucchini Boats (Chapter 13)

Saturday
Breakfast: Bacon, Kale, and Sun-Dried Tomato Quiche (Chapter 8)
Lunch: Leftover Moroccan Chicken Tagine
Dinner: Yellow Pepper and Tomato Soup with Basil topped with Fresh Gluten-Free Croutons
(Chapters 11 and 12)
Dessert: Baked Stuffed Apples (Chapter 18)
Snack: Crunchy Snack Mix (Chapter 13)

Week 3:

Sunday
Breakfast: Frittata with Asparagus, Cheddar, and Monterey Jack (Chapter 8)
Lunch: Grilled Pork and Mango Salsa Sandwich (Chapter 8)
Dinner: Thai Chicken with Peanut Dipping Sauce and Egg Drop Soup with Ginger and Lemon
(Chapters 8 and 11)
Dessert: Dark Chocolate, Walnut, and Hazelnut Torte (Chapter 18)
Snack: Chili Bean Dip with Dipping Vegetables (Chapter 13)

Monday
Breakfast: Cottage Cheese Pancakes (Chapter 7)
Lunch: Indian Vegetable Cakes (Chapter 8)
Dinner: Leftover Frittata with Asparagus, Cheddar, and Monterey Jack and 1 cup mixed greens
with 2 tablespoons Lemon Pepper Dressing (Chapter 12)
Dessert: Peaches 'n' Cream Smoothie (Chapter 14)
Snack: ¼ cup walnuts

Tuesday
Breakfast: Herbed Vegetable Omelet (Chapter 7)
Lunch: Cashew-Zucchini Soup with Sweet Corn Bread (Chapters 11 and 10)
Dinner: Egyptian Lentils and Rice (Chapter 16)
Dessert: Leftover Dark Chocolate, Walnut, and Hazelnut Torte
Snack: Roasted Sweet and Spicy Soybeans (Chapter 13)

Wednesday
Breakfast: Irish Oatmeal and Poached Fruit (Chapter 7)
Lunch: Chicken Breast with Scallions, Snap Peas, and Beans (Chapter 8)
Dinner: Golden Sautéed Diver Scallops with Classic Italian Risotto (Chapters 9 and 10)
Dessert: Berry Banana Smoothie (Chapter 14)
Snack: Leftover Roasted Sweet and Spicy Soybeans

Thursday

Breakfast: 2 scrambled eggs with 1 cup mixed berries
Lunch: Spiced Stuffed Peppers (Chapter 8)
Dinner: Beef and Sweet Potato Stew (Chapter 11)
Dessert: Nut-Crusted Key Lime Pie (Chapter 18)
Snack: Cranberry Apple Juice (Chapter 15) with 1 cup sliced celery

Friday

Breakfast: 1 cup Greek yogurt topped with ¼ cup almonds
Lunch: Smooth Cauliflower Soup with Coriander (Chapter 16)
Dinner: Étoufée (Chapter 17)
Dessert: Blueberry-Peach Cobbler (Chapter 18)
Snack: Sliced cucumbers topped with Tomatillo Salsa (Chapter 13)

Saturday

Breakfast: Shirred Eggs with Crumbled Cheddar Topping (Chapter 7)
Lunch: Leftover Smooth Cauliflower Soup with Coriander
Dinner: Beef Tenderloin with Chimichurri (Chapter 9)
Dessert: Leftover Nut-Crusted Key Lime Pie
Snack: Tex-Mex Taco Dip (Chapter 13) and 1 cup sliced vegetables

Week 4:

Sunday
Breakfast: Bacon, Kale, and Sun-Dried Tomato Quiche (Chapter 8)
Lunch: Grilled Vegetable and Cheese Panini (Chapter 8)
Dinner: Stuffed Eggplant with Ricotta and Spices (Chapter 9)
Dessert: Cranberry Pear Compote (Chapter 17) over ½ cup ice cream
Snack: Fruit Skewers with Yogurt Dip (Chapter 13)

Monday
Breakfast: Scrambled Eggs with Sausage and Jalapeño (Chapter 7)
Lunch: White Bean Ratatouille (Chapter 10)
Dinner: Leftover Bacon, Kale, and Sun-Dried Tomato Quiche
Dessert: Brie-Stuffed Celery with Walnuts (Chapter 13)
Snack: Leftover Cranberry Pear Compote and 1 cup plain yogurt

Tuesday
Breakfast: Strawberry Pancakes (Chapter 7)
Lunch: New England Clam Chowder (Chapter 11)
Dinner: Rosemary Pork Chops with Apples and Raisins (Chapter 9)
Dessert: Pear and Ginger Smoothie (Chapter 14)
Snack: Spicy Guacamole (Chapter 13) with 1 cup grape tomatoes

Wednesday
Breakfast: Egg-and-Cheese-Stuffed Tomatoes (Chapter 7)
Lunch: Cashew-Zucchini Soup (Chapter 11)
Dinner: Spicy Asian Salad with Grilled Tuna (Chapter 12)
Dessert: Simple Berry Crumble (Chapter 18)
Snack: Amazing Avocado Smoothie (Chapter 14)

Thursday

Breakfast: Blackberry Lemon Smoothie (Chapter 14)

Lunch: Broccoli Soup with Cheddar (Chapter 11)

Dinner: Baked Mushroom and Fontina Risotto (Chapter 10) with 1 cup mixed greens, topped with 2 tablespoons Italian Dressing (Chapter 12)

Dessert: Baked Stuffed Apples (Chapter 18)

Snack: Pickled Mushrooms (Chapter 16)

Friday

Breakfast: Chestnut Flour Crepes (Chapter 7)

Lunch: Vegan Chili (Chapter 16)

Dinner: Curried Shrimp with Avocados (Chapter 9)

Dessert: Leftover Simple Berry Crumble

Snack: Spiced Pecans (Chapter 16)

Saturday

Breakfast: Spinach and Gorgonzola Egg-White Omelet (Chapter 7)

Lunch: Southwestern Bean Salad (Chapter 10)

Dinner: Poached Chicken with Pears and Herbs and Spinach and Tomato Sauté (Chapters 9 and 16)

Dessert: Cocoa Banana Smoothie (Chapter 14)

Snack: 1 cup leftover Vegan Chili

APPENDIX B

Sources

Chapter 2

Austin, G.L., et al. "A Very Low-Carbohydrate Diet Improves Gastroesophageal Reflux and Its Symptoms." *Digestive Diseases and Sciences* 51, no. 8 (2006): 1307–12.

Becker, D.J., et al. "A Comparison of High and Low Fat Meals on Postprandial Esophageal Acid Exposure." *American Journal of Gastroenterology* 84, no. 7 (1989): 782–86.

Boekema, P.J., et al. "Coffee and Gastrointestinal Function: Facts and Fiction; A Review." *Scandinavian Journal of Gastroenterology* 34, no. 230 (1999): 35–39.

Bujanda, L. "The Effects of Alcohol Consumption upon the Gastrointestinal Tract." *American Journal of Gastroenterology* 95, no. 12 (2000): 3374–82.

Cuomo, A., et al. "Reflux Oesophagitis in Adult Celiac Disease: Beneficial Effect of a Gluten Free Diet." *Gut* 52, no. 4 (2003): 514–17.

El-Serag, H.B., et al. "Dietary Intake and the Risk of Gastro-oesophageal Reflux Disease: A Cross-Sectional Study in Volunteers." *Gut* 54, no. 1 (2005): 11–17.

Hamoui, N., et al. "Response of the Lower Esophageal Sphincter to Gastric Distention by Carbonated Beverages." *Journal of Gastrointestinal Surgery* 10, no. 6 (2006): 870–77.

Iwakiri, K., et al. "Relationship Between Postprandial Esophageal Acid Exposure and Meal Volume and Fat Content." *Digestive Diseases and Sciences* 41, no. 5 (1996): 926–30.

Jiao, L., et al. "Dietary Intake of Vegetables, Folate, and Antioxidants and the Risk of Barrett's Esophagus." *Cancer Causes and Control* 24, no. 5 (2013): 1005–14.

Johnson, T., et al. "Systematic Review: The Effects of Carbonated Beverages on Gastro-oesophageal Reflux Disease." *Alimentary Pharmacology and Therapeutics* 1, no. 6 (2010): 607–14.

Kubo, A., et al. "Dietary Antioxidants, Fruits and Vegetables, and the Risk of Barrett's Esophagus." *American Journal of Gastroenterology* 103, no. 7 (2008): 1614–24.

Lucendo, A.J. "Esophageal Manifestations of Celiac Disease." *Diseases of the Esophagus* 24, no. 7 (2011): 470–75.

Lukić, M., et al. "The Impact of the Vitamins A, C, and E in the Prevention of Gastroesophageal Reflux Disease, Barrett's Oesophagus and Oesophageal Adenocarcinoma." *Collegium Antropologicum* 36, no. 3 (2012): 867–72.

Nachman, F., et al. "Gastroesophageal Reflux Symptoms in Patients with Celiac Disease and the Effects of a Gluten-Free Diet." *Clinical Gastroenterology and Hepatology* 9, no. 3 (2011): 214–19.

Nilsson, M., et al. "Lifestyle Related Risk Factors in the Aetiology of Gastro-oesophageal Reflux." *Gut* 53, no. 12 (2004): 1730–35.

Schuppan, D., et al. "Celiac Disease: From Pathogenesis to Novel Therapies." *Gastroenterology* 137, no. 6 (2009): 1912–33.

Steevens, J., et al. "Vegetables and Fruits Consumption and Risk of Esophageal and Gastric Acid Cancer Subtypes in the Netherlands Cohort Study." *International Journal of Cancer* 129, no. 11 (2011): 2681–93.

Usai, P., et al. "Effect of a Gluten-Free Diet on Preventing Recurrence of Gastroesophageal Reflux Disease–Related Symptoms in Adult Celiac Patients with Nonerosive Reflux Disease." *Journal of Gastroenterology and Hepatology* 23, no. 9 (2008): 1368–72.

Yancy, W.S., "Improvement of Gastroesophageal Reflux Disease after Initiation of a low-Carbohydrate Diet: Five Brief Case Reports." *Alternative Therapies in Health and Medicine* 7, no. 6 (2001): 116–19.

Yancy, W.S., et al. "A Low-Carbohydrate, Ketogenic Diet versus a Low-Fat Diet to Treat Obesity and Hyperlipidemia: A Randomized, Controlled Trial." *Annals of Internal Medicine* 140, no. 10 (2004): 769–77.

Chapter 3

Aucoin, M., et al. "Mindfulness-Based Therapies in the Treatment of Functional Gastrointestinal Disorders: A Meta-Analysis." *Evidence-Based Complementary and Alternative Therapies* 2014 (2014): 1–11.

Cook, M.B., et al. "Cigarette Smoking Increases Risks of Barrett's Esophagus: An Analysis of the Barrett's and Esophageal Adenocarcinoma Consortium." *Gastroenterology* 142, no. 4 (2012): 744–53.

Djärv, T., et al. "Physical Activity, Obesity and Gastroesophageal Reflux Disease in the General Population." *World Journal of Gastroenterology* 18, no. 28 (2012): 3710–14.

El-Serag, H., "The Association Between Obesity and GERD: A Review of the Epidemiological Evidence." *Digestive Diseases and Sciences* 53, no. 9 (2008): 2307–12.

El-Serag, H., et al. "Obesity Is an Independent Risk Factor for GERD Symptoms and Erosive Gastritis." *American Journal of Gastroenterology* 100, no. 6 (2005): 1243–50.

Faramarzi, M., et al. "A Randomized Controlled Trial of Brief Psychoanalytic Psychotherapy in Patients with Functional Dyspepsia." *Asian Jour of Psychiatry* 6, no. 3 (2013): 228–34.

Fraser-Moodie, C.A., et al. "Weight Loss Has an Independent Beneficial Effect on Symptoms of

Gastrooesophageal Reflux in Patients Who Are Overweight." *Scandinavian Journal of Gastroenterology* 34., no. 4 (1999): 337–40.

Fujiwara, Y., et al. "Cigarette Smoking and Its Association with Overlapping Gastroesophageal Reflux Disease, Functional Dyspepsia, or Irritable Bowel Syndrome." *Internal Medicine* 50, no. 21 (2011): 2443–47.

Godsey, J. "The Role of Mindfulness Based Interventions in the Treatment of Obesity and Eating Disorders: An Integrative Review." *Complementary Therapies in Medicine* 21, no. 4 (2013): 430–39.

Hamilton, J., et al. "A Randomized Controlled Trial of Psychotherapy in Patients with Chronic Functional Dyspepsia." *Gastroenterology* 119, no. 3 (2000): 661–69.

Hardikar, S., et al. "The Role of Tobacco, Alcohol, and Obesity in Neoplastic Progression to Esophageal Adenocarcinoma: A Prospective Study of Barrett's Esophagus." *PLOS One* 8, no. 1 (2013): 1–9.

Jansson, C., et al. "Stressful Psychosocial Factors and Symptoms of Gastroesophageal Reflux Disease: A Population-Based Study in Norway." *Scandinavian Journal of Gastroenterology* 45, no. 1 (2010): 21–29.

Kahrilas, P.J., and R.R. Gupta. "Mechanisms of Acid Reflux Associated with Cigarette Smoking." *Gut* 31, no. 1 (1990): 4–10.

Konturek, P.C., et al. "Stress and the Gut: Pathophysiology, Clinical Consequences, Diagnostic Approach and Treatment Options." *Journal of Physiology and Pharmacology* 62, no. 6 (2011): 591–99.

Ledikwe, J.H., et al. "Portion Sizes and the Obesity Epidemic." *Journal of Nutrition* 135, no. 4 (2005): 905–909.

Ness-Jensen, E., at al. "Weight Loss and Reduction in Gastroesophageal Reflux: A Prospective Population-Based Cohort Study; The HUNT Study." *American Journal of Gastroenterology* 108, no. 3 (2013): 376–82.

Ness-Jensen, E., et al. "Tobacco Smoking Cessation and Improved Gastroesophageal Reflux: A Prospective Population-Based Cohort Study; The HUNT Study." *American Journal of Gastroenterology* 104, no. 2 (2014): 171–77.

Nilsson, M., et al. "Lifestyle Related Risk Factors in the Aetiology of Gastro-esophageal Reflux." *Gut* 53, no. 12 (2004): 1730–35.

Singh, M., et al. "Weight Loss Can Lead to Resolution of Gastroesophageal Reflux Disease Symptoms: A Prospective Intervention Trial." *Obesity* 21, no. 2 (2013): 284–90.

Smit, C.F., et al. "Effect of Cigarette Smoking on Gastropharyngeal and Gastroesophageal

Reflux." *Annals of Otology, Rhinology, and Laryngology* 110, no. 2 (2001): 190–93.

Yates, M., et al. "Body Mass Index, Smoking, and Alcohol and Risks of Barrett's Esophagus and Esophageal Adenocarcinoma: A UK Prospective Cohort Study." *Digestive Diseases and Sciences* 59, no. 7 (2014): 1552–59.

Chapter 4

Aseeri, M., et al. "Gastric Acid Suppression by Proton Pump Inhibitors as a Risk Factor for *Clostridium Difficile*–Associated Diarrhea in Hospitalized Patients." *American Journal of Gastroenterology* 103, no. 9 (2008): 2308–13.

Hershcovici, T., and R. Fass. "Pharmacological Management of GERD: Where Does It Stand Now?" *Trends in Pharmacological Sciences* 32, no. 4 (2011): 258–64.

Lam, J.R., et al. "Proton Pump Inhibitors and Histamine 2 Receptor Antagonist Use and Vitamin B_{12} Deficiency." *Journal of the American Medical Association* 310, no. 22 (2013): 2435–42.

Lau, Y.T., and N.N. Ahmed. "Fracture Risk and Bone Mineral Density Reduction Associated with Proton Pump Inhibitors." *Pharmacotherapy* 32, no. 1 (2012): 67–79.

Leontiadis, G.I., and P. Moayyedi. "Proton Pump Inhibitors and Risk of Bone Fractures." *Current Treatment Options in Gastroenterology* 12, no. 4 (2014): 414–23.

Mandel, K.G., et al. "Review Article: Alginate-Raft Formulations in the Treatment of Heartburn and Acid Reflux." *Alimentary Pharmacology and Therapeutics* 14, no. 6 (2000): 669–90.

McRorie, J.W., et al. "Evidence-Based Treatment of Frequent Heartburn: The Benefits and Limitations of Over-the-Counter Medications." *Journal of the American Association of Nurse Practitioners* 26, no. 6 (2014): 330–39.

n.a., "Proton Pump Inhibitors: Bacterial Pneumonia." *Prescrire International* 21, no. 130 (2012): 210–12.

Quartarone, G. "Gastroesophageal Reflux in Pregnancy: A Systematic Review on the Benefit of Raft-Forming Agents." *Minerva Ginecologica* 65, no. 5 (2013): 541–49.

Wang, Y.-K., et al. "Current Pharmacological Management of Gastro-esophageal Reflux Disease." *Gastroenterology Research and Practice* 2013 (2013): 1–12.

Zerbib, F. "Medical Treatment of GORD: Emerging Therapeutic Targets and Concepts." *Best Practice and Research: Clinical Gastroenterology* 24, no. 6 (2010): 937–46.

Chapter 5

Aly, A.M., et al. "Licorice: A Possible Anti-inflammatory and Anti-ulcer Drug." *AAPS PharmSciTech* 6, no. 1 (2005): 74–82.

Brown, R., et al. "Effect of GutsyGum™, a Novel Gum on Subjective Ratings of Gastroesophageal Reflux Following a Refluxogenic Meal." *Journal of Dietary Supplements* 21 August 2014: online publication.

Calvert, E.L., et al. "Long-Term Improvement in Functional Dyspepsia Using Hypnotherapy." *Gastroenterology* 123, no. 6 (2002): 1778–85.

Dickman, R., et al. "Clinical Trial: Acupuncture vs. Doubling the Proton Pump Inhibitor Dose in Refractory Heartburn." *Alimentary Pharmacology and Therapeutics* 26, no. 10 (2007): 1333–44.

Holtmann, G., et al. "Efficacy of Artichoke Leaf Extract in the Treatment of Patients with Functional Dyspepsia: A Six-Week Placebo-Controlled Double-Blind Multicentre Trial." *Alimentary Pharmacology and Therapeutics* 18, nos. 11–12 (2003): 1099–105.

Kandil, T.S., et al. "The Potential Therapeutic Effect of Melatonin in Gastro-Esophageal Reflux Disease." *BMC Gastroenterology* 10, no. 7 (2010): 1–9.

Konturek, P.C., et al. "Esophagoprotection Mediated by Exogenous and Endogenous Melatonin in an Experimental Model of Reflux Esophagitis." *Journal of Pineal Research* 55, no. 1 (2013): 46–57.

Konturek, P.C., et al. "Stress and the Gut: Pathophysiology, Clinical Consequences, Diagnostic Approach and Treatment Options." *Journal of Physiology and Pharmacology* 62, no. 6 (2001): 591–99.

May, B., et al. "Efficacy and Tolerability of a Fixed Combination of Peppermint Oil and Caraway Oil in Patients Suffering from Functional Dyspepsia." *Alimentary Pharmacology and Therapeutics* 14, no. 12 (2000): 1671–77.

Mukherjee, M., et al. "Anti-ulcer and Antioxidant Activity of GutGuard." *Indian Journal of Experimental Biology* 48, no. 3 (2010): 269–74.

Patrick, L. "Gastroesophageal Reflux Disease (GERD): A Review of Conventional and Alternative Treatments." *Alternative Medicine Review* 16, no. 2 (2011): 116–33.

Pereira, R. "Regression of Gastroesophageal Reflux Disease Symptoms Using Dietary Supplementation with Melatonin, Vitamins and Amino Acids: Comparison with Omeprazole." *Journal of Pineal Research* 41, no. 3 (2006): 195–200.

Rafiee, P., et al. "Effect of Curcumin on Acidic pH-Induced Expression of IL-6 and IL-8 in Human Esophageal Epithelial Cells (HET-1A): Role of PKC, MAPKs, and NF-kappaB." *American Journal of Physiology: Gastrointestinal and Liver Physiology* 296, no. 2 (2009): 388–98.

Stacher, G., et al. "Effect of Hypnotic Suggestion of Relaxation on Basal and Betazole-Stimulated Gastric Acid Secretion." *Gastroenterology* 68, no. 4 (1974): 656–61.

Sun, J. "D-Limonene: Safety and Clinical Applications." *Alternative Medicine Review* 12, no. 3 (2007): 259–64.

Thavorn, K., et al. "Efficacy of Turmeric in the Treatment of Digestive Disorders: A Systematic Review and Meta-Analysis Protocol." *Systematic Reviews* 3, no. 71 (2014): 2–6.

Zhang, C.X., et al. "Clinical Study on the Treatment of Gastroesophageal Reflux by Acupuncture." *Chinese Journal of Integrative Medicine* 16, no. 4 (2010): 298–303.

Chapter 6

De Groot, N.L., et al. "Systematic Review: The Effects of Conservative and Surgical Treatment for Obesity on Gastro-Oesophageal Reflux Disease." *Alimentary Pharmacology and Therapeutics* 30, nos. 11–12 (2009): 1091–102.

DeVault, K.R., and D.O. Castell. "Updated Guidelines for the Diagnosis and Treatment of Gastroesophageal Reflux Disease." *American Journal of Gastroenterology* 94, no. 6 (1999): 1434–42.

El-Hadi, M., et al. "The Effect of Bariatric Surgery on Gastroesophageal Reflux Disease." *Canadian Journal of Surgery* 57, no. 2 (2014): 139–44.

n.a., "Guidelines for Surgical Treatment of Gastroesophageal Reflux Disease (GERD)." *Surgical Endoscopy* 12, no. 2 (1998): 186–88.

Rodriguez, L., et al. "Long-Term Results of Electrical Stimulation of the Lower Esophageal Sphincter for the Treatment of Gastroesophageal Reflux Disease." *Endoscopy* 45, no. 8 (2013): 596–604.

Trad, K.S., et al. "Transoral Incisionless Fundoplication Effective in Eliminating GERD Symptoms in Partial Responders to Proton Pump Inhibitor Therapy at 6 Months." *Surgical Innovation* 21 April 2014: online publication.

Zhi, X.T., et al. "Management of Gastroesophageal Reflux Disease: Medications, Surgery, or Endoscopic Therapy?" *Journal of Long-Term Effects of Medical Implants* 15, no. 4 (2005): 375–88.

Standard U.S./Metric Measurement Conversions

VOLUME CONVERSIONS

U.S. Volume Measure	Metric Equivalent
⅛ teaspoon	0.5 milliliter
¼ teaspoon	1 milliliter
½ teaspoon	2 milliliters
1 teaspoon	5 milliliters
½ tablespoon	7 milliliters
1 tablespoon (3 teaspoons)	15 milliliters
2 tablespoons (1 fluid ounce)	30 milliliters
¼ cup (4 tablespoons)	60 milliliters
⅓ cup	90 milliliters
½ cup (4 fluid ounces)	125 milliliters
⅔ cup	160 milliliters
¾ cup (6 fluid ounces)	180 milliliters
1 cup (16 tablespoons)	250 milliliters
1 pint (2 cups)	500 milliliters
1 quart (4 cups)	1 liter (about)

WEIGHT CONVERSIONS

U.S. Weight Measure	Metric Equivalent
½ ounce	15 grams
1 ounce	30 grams
2 ounces	60 grams
3 ounces	85 grams
¼ pound (4 ounces)	115 grams
½ pound (8 ounces)	225 grams
¾ pound (12 ounces)	340 grams
1 pound (16 ounces)	454 grams

OVEN TEMPERATURE CONVERSIONS

Degrees Fahrenheit	Degrees Celsius
200 degrees F	95 degrees C
250 degrees F	120 degrees C
275 degrees F	135 degrees C
300 degrees F	150 degrees C
325 degrees F	160 degrees C
350 degrees F	180 degrees C
375 degrees F	190 degrees C
400 degrees F	205 degrees C
425 degrees F	220 degrees C
450 degrees F	230 degrees C

BAKING PAN SIZES

American	Metric
8 x 1½ inch round baking pan	20 x 4 cm cake tin
9 x 1½ inch round baking pan	23 x 3.5 cm cake tin
11 x 7 x 1½ inch baking pan	28 x 18 x 4 cm baking tin
13 x 9 x 2 inch baking pan	30 x 20 x 5 cm baking tin
2 quart rectangular baking dish	30 x 20 x 3 cm baking tin
15 x 10 x 2 inch baking pan	30 x 25 x 2 cm baking tin (Swiss roll tin)
9 inch pie plate	22 x 4 or 23 x 4 cm pie plate
7 or 8 inch springform pan	18 or 20 cm springform or loose bottom cake tin
9 x 5 x 3 inch loaf pan	23 x 13 x 7 cm or 2 lb narrow loaf or pate tin
1½ quart casserole	1.5 liter casserole
2 quart casserole	2 liter casserole

Index